SILENT RISK

SILENT RISK

Issues about the Human Umbilical Cord

Jason H. Collins, MD, MSCR

Copyright © 2014 by Jason H. Collins, MD, MSCR.

Library of Congress Control Number:		2014911209
ISBN:	Hardcover	978-1-4990-3910-8
	Softcover	978-1-4990-3911-5
	eBook	978-1-4990-3909-2

All rights reserved. No part of this book may be reproduced or transmitted in any form or by any means, electronic or mechanical, including photocopying, recording, or by any information storage and retrieval system, without permission in writing from the copyright owner.

Any people depicted in stock imagery provided by Thinkstock are models, and such images are being used for illustrative purposes only.
Certain stock imagery © Thinkstock.

This book was printed in the United States of America.

Rev. date: 06/28/2014

To order additional copies of this book, contact:
Xlibris LLC
1-888-795-4274
www.Xlibris.com
Orders@Xlibris.com
552844

CONTENTS

Preface 7
Acknowledgments 9
Introduction 13

Chapter One: Origin and Development of the Umbilical Cord.. 19
Chapter Two: The Umbilical Cord: The Problems of
                 Supply and Demand 43
Chapter Three: Fetal Behavior and Physiology 64
Chapter Four: What Animal Research Teaches Us about
                 Umbilical Cord Accidents 79
Chapter Five: Management of Umbilical Cord Anomalies,
                 Abnormalities, and Complications 90
Chapter Six: The Future of Umbilical Cord Research 102

Recommended Reading 121

PREFACE

Congenital abnormalities of the human umbilical cord and placenta may result in significant complications during labour. The ill-effects are predominantly upon the newborn-less common maternal morbidity and mortality may result.
—Albert A. Earn, MD, MSc
Winnipeg, Canada 1951

The issue of umbilical cord-related fetal harm and fetal stillbirth is unaddressed in modern reproductive care. Although observations of umbilical cord-related deaths have not necessarily proven causation, it is difficult not to ask, what is the relationship? It is time to answer this question and to discern the full ramifications of umbilical cord-related injury and death. The information discussed here is based on twenty-five years of research and a review of medical journals and texts. The authors have searched over one thousand peer-reviewed articles published as of 1950 to provide a current panorama of this reproductive problem, which is not limited to humans. In addition, the Pregnancy Institute is dedicated to solving the problem of umbilical cord accidents. The Pregnancy Institute is a 501(c)(3) nonprofit medical research corporation cofounded by Jason H. Collins, MD, MSCR, an obstetrician interested in improving birth outcomes; Charles L. Collins, BSE, MD, a pathologist interested in placental changes; and Candace C. Collins, MD, a pediatric ophthalmologist interested in learning disabilities. By assembling this story, it is our goal to persuade other researchers to turn their attention to the problem of solving umbilical cord accidents and anomalies. Hopefully, the future will see a permanent solution. The mother, also, can play a role in solving the tragedy of umbilical cord accidents. While it is unknown how much time is needed for a fetus to die, it is believed that some fetuses die slowly.

Fetal behavior is consistent and can have a repetitive (circadian) rhythm. As discussed later, awareness of fetal movements, sleep-wake cycles, and tendencies may provide an initial warning of a compromised fetus. Verbalizing these changes to the obstetrician may alert everyone of the need for a closer look at the fetus with ultrasound and fetal monitoring. We hope that after reading this book, you, the reader, will have a greater understanding of this tragedy. The expectant mother will hopefully understand her role in solving this tragedy, and the medical professional will realize their responsibility to protect the baby from UCA.

ACKNOWLEDGMENTS

We would like to thank the patients who provided us with the need to find a solution to the problem of umbilical cord accidents. Many parents courageously came forward and shared with us their experiences of umbilical cord-related stillbirth. To discuss these events is difficult for them because to lose a normal fetus is so unique an experience.

Many scientists, researchers, physicians, midwives, and nurses over the years have grappled with this issue. One who stands out in modern times is Jason C. Birnholz, MD, who summarized the issue of the supply line (umbilical cord). In the context of an overall vision he states:

> The practical goal of clinical obstetrics is to deliver an infant who will not only survive but develop without handicap from a prenatal or perinatal insult. (Birnholz 1990)

This goal requires the application of tools called ultrasonography and fetal heart rate monitoring. Because of the efforts of Dr. Douglas Howry and Dr. John J. Wild, we can view the fetus in the uterus. Thanks to Dr. Edward H. Hon, fetal heart rate monitoring became established in obstetrical care. Many individuals have added to these great works and continue to do so today. Now, many differing opinions exist about how effective these tools have been to reproductive care and outcomes. Let there be no mistake—to view the fetus and assess its physiology offers a chance to save a dying fetus where otherwise there would be no chance. Many thanks go to Tulane University Medical Library whose holdings of journals, texts, and special collections offer a repository of knowledge covering two hundred years of obstetrical medicine. Margaret Verzwyvelt, Patsy Copeland, and Cathleen Furlong provided much valuable time retrieving articles and hunting down rare interlibrary loans. Thank you to Mr. W. Postel for allowing the many unusual requests to hold his books at home for weeks. Lastly, thank you to Jeanette Beauman, the executive secretary of the Pregnancy Institute, who typed everything, mailed everything, and did everything to bring this book to reality. Thank you to Patricia Taylor, who donated her editorial expertise and believed in the book.

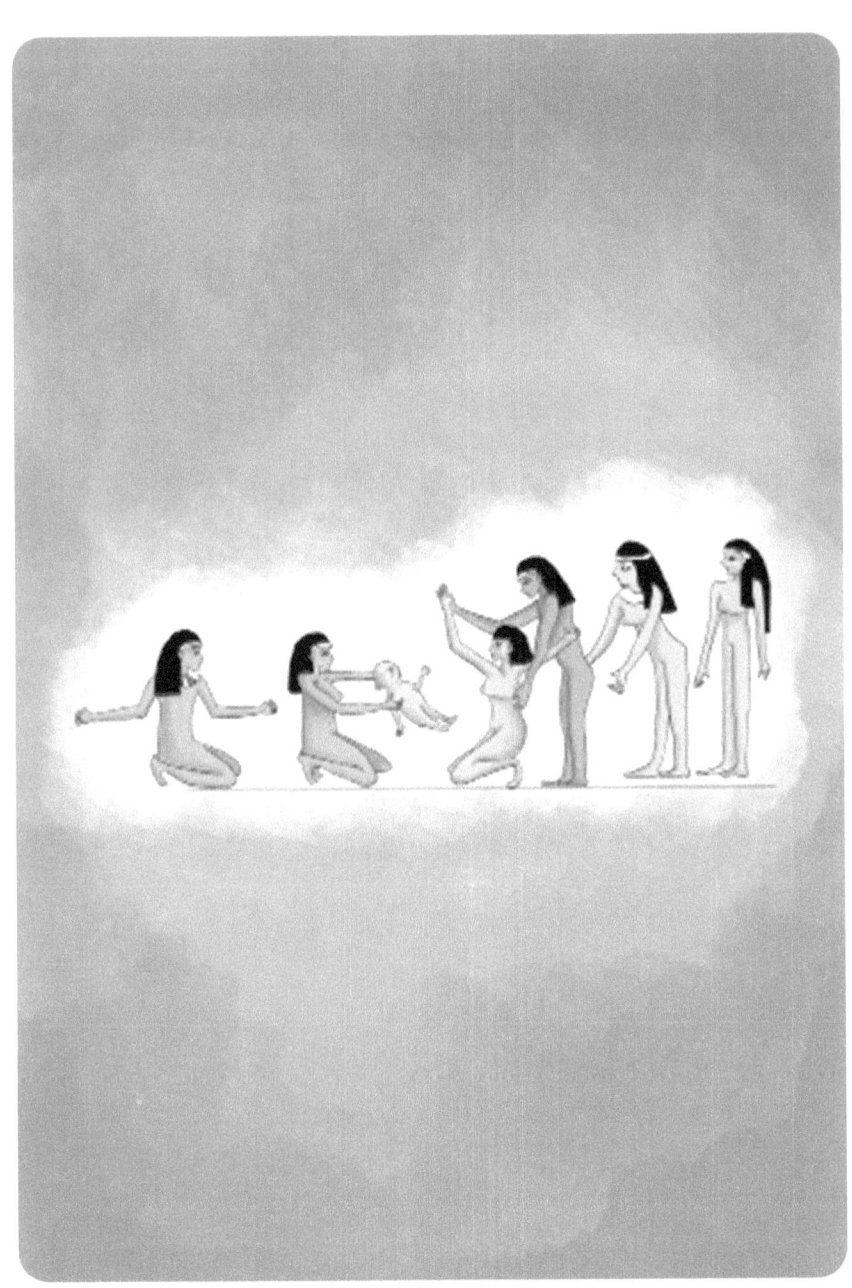

Cleopatra's Birth

INTRODUCTION

A survey of a number of British and American textbooks has yielded scant information on this subject [of umbilical cord complications].
—Kan Pun Shui, BS, MB, and
Nickolson J. Eastman, MD
Hong Kong
1956

It has always been a surprise to me that so little comment has been made on the large proportion of stillbirths which is associated with one or other of the various cord complications.
—T. F. Corkill, MD
Wellington General Hospital
New Zealand
1961

The umbilical cord is an ancient structure which has many functions. Melbourne Museum has a 375 million year old placoderm fish fossil showing an embryo attached to its mother by an umbilical cord (*http://museumvictoria.com.au/learning-federation/video-temp/mother-fish/mother-fish-video/*).

Umbilical cord events occur in all mammals. From dolphins to rodents to elephants to horses,the umbilical cord is essential for life. If the umbilical cord structure fails the fetus will be stillborn.

Recommended Reading

Recurrent umbilical cord accidents in a bottlenose dolphin Tursiops truncates. Daniel García-Párraga, Fiona Brook, José

Luís Crespo-Picazo, Teresa Álvaro, Mónica Valls, Mariola Penadés, Joaquín Ortega, Juan Manuel Corpa. DISEASES OF AQUATIC ORGANISMS Vol. 108: 177–180, 2014 doi: 10.3354/dao02711

One has to wonder what thoughts prehistoric humans had when confronted with the stillbirth of a baby entangled in its umbilical cord.

Egyptian history suggests the placenta with its cord was needed at death to be buried and was kept and stored from birth. Two mummified babies were found in Tutankhamen's tomb and were thought to be stillbirths. No mummified placental or cord remains have been seen.

Some insights from more recent times suggest the umbilical cord represented an omen, a sacred talisman, predictor of future fertility. In Europe, Australia, Africa, and Americas, the umbilical cord was dried and soaked in water for consumption to ensure future fertility. It was eaten, hung from tree branches, and stuffed in volcanic rock crevices at sites such as the Birthing Stones in Kukahiioko, Oahu. In Turkey and Japan, the umbilical cord is preserved. In Japan, there is a special box called *kotobuki bako* in which is preserved a segment of the umbilical cord for future good fortune. Recently a preserved 77 year old umbilical cord underwent DNA analysis to determine paternal origins of a japanese family.

Chinese literature suggests the cord has medicinal properties. European insights beginning with Galen (AD 129-200) suggested the umbilical cord served to nurture the fetus through arteries and veins. Leonardo da Vinci (1452-1519) observed that the cord was as long as the fetus at a given gestational age. Spiglius (1631) determined blood flow direction, and Harvey (1657) suggested that interruption of this blood flow could be the cause of fetal death if the cord was compressed. Early descriptions of fetal loss from cord entanglement date as far back as three hundred years ago.

In 1750, the British obstetrician William Smellie describes case number 172 in his *Treatise on the Theory and Practice of Midwifery* as a stillborn with four cord loops around the neck. One of the first published drawings of an UCA was by Andrew Bell in the *Encyclopedia Britannica*

(1769), depicting a fetal death with a combination of one nuchal cord, a body loop, and a true knot (currently on the cover of the Royal College of Obstetricians and Gynaecologists [UK] brochure). By the 1800s, many observations were recorded of distressed fetuses born with cord entanglement and cord abnormalities. UCA was established as a definite cause of stillbirth. Over the last twenty years, images of four cord loops similar to Dr. Smellie's description and management of entangled babies have been peer reviewed and published in medical journals, demonstrating stillbirth can be avoided.

A review of these early descriptions suggest *clinical symptoms* such as pulling sensations felt at the top of the uterus and excessive fetal movement (hyperactivity) followed by decreased fetal activity prior to fetal death. Today, the field of obstetrics is confronted with the issue of umbilical cord complications—a timeless, almost prehistoric example of how imperfect reproductive evolution sometimes can be. Issues of birth-related blood loss, infection, and surgical intervention (C-section) have matured. Premature birth, congenital anomalies, and toxemia still challenge the obstetrical community. Because umbilical cord accidents may represent a small number of fetal deaths, the motivation to investigate this reproductive tragedy may not be seen as urgent. However, out of four million births per year in the United States, an estimated eight thousand umbilical cord-related deaths occur. This is known as mortality. What harm occurs to the live-born fetus due to an umbilical cord complication is unknown. Obstetrical scientists call this harm morbidity. This morbidity is studied in terms of delivery outcome—meaning, what harm is noticeable and how much. This harm often goes unnoticed for years. What harm does occur is rarely recorded. Prenatal umbilical cord compression is currently suspected to provide such morbidity as neurologic and cardiac damage and may be as subtle as mild learning disabilities or as obvious as cerebral palsy. This is currently considered speculative by most, but not all, reproductive scientists. The Perinatal Umbilical Cord Project (PUCP), an ongoing project at the Pregnancy Institute, seeks to understand the issue of umbilical cord complications, an event particularly tragic to the mother. If mothers are to be comforted, an explanation of how these events happen is important. The PUCP has established a scientific method (protocol) of observation and has prospectively inspected over one thousand pregnancy cases. Method: All patients receive standard prenatal care starting with an exam at eight to ten weeks. This includes a vaginal ultrasound, a second ultrasound at twenty weeks, and a third ultrasound study at twenty-eight weeks screens for umbilical cord problems. Also, at every visit, the fetal heart rate is studied for ten to fifteen minutes and recorded. Patients identified with umbilical cord abnormalities (UCA) are watched biweekly. Repeat studies with ultrasound and fetal heart rate monitoring occur as needed.

"Umbilical cord abnormalities accounted for 10% of our possible or probable causes of death, which is considerably higher than in previous studies, and were more common in stillbirths of greater than 32 weeks gestation…As a potentially preventable cause of stillbirth, cord abnormalities deserve further investigation ".The Stillbirth Collaborative Research Network Writing Group JAMA, December 14, 2011—Vol 306, No. 22; pg **2466.**

As evidence and data accumulate, the authors hope that a solution can be created that will allow successful management of the normal pregnancy threatened by an umbilical cord complication.

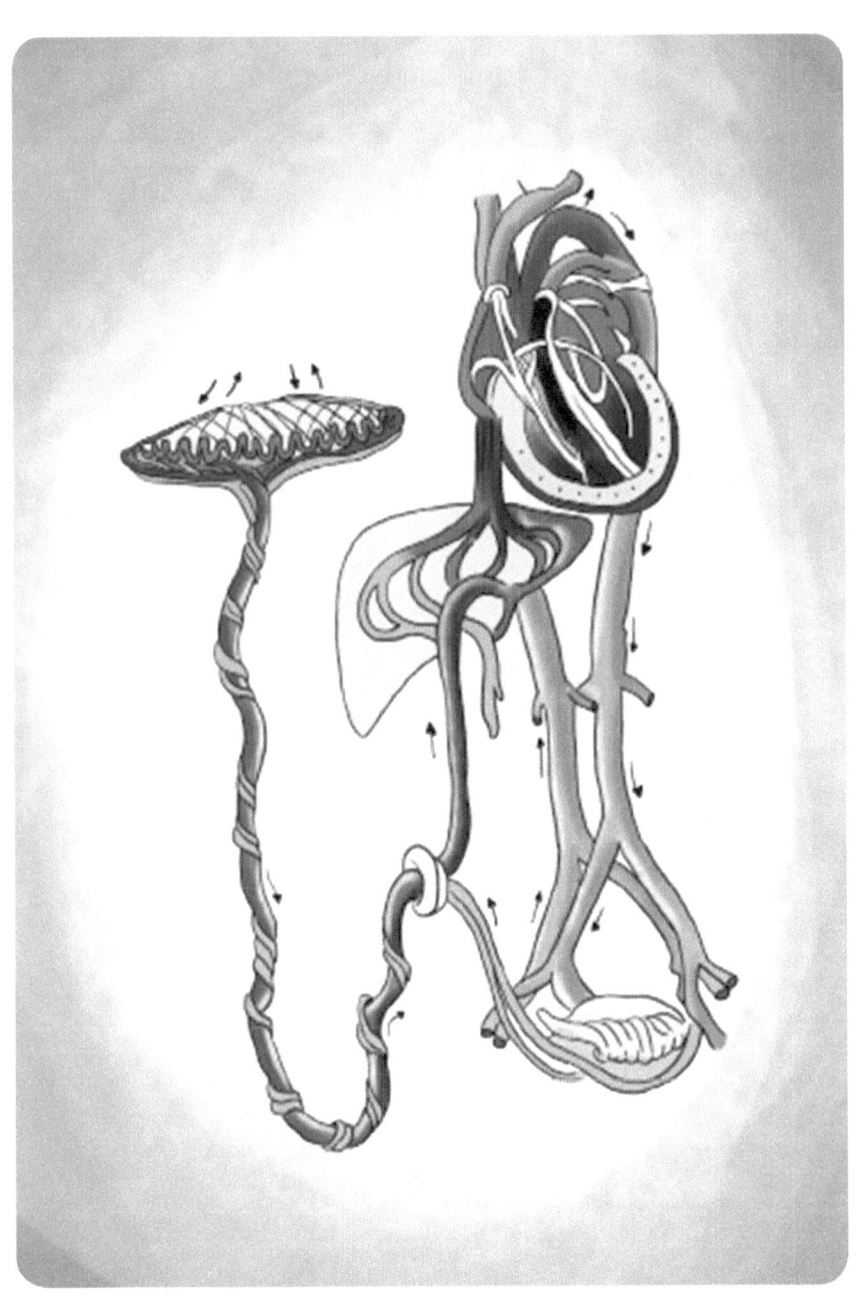

Placental Umbilical Circulation

CHAPTER ONE

Origin and Development of the Umbilical Cord

The human blastocyst implants into uterine decidua . . . There is little realization that this supreme accomplishment is the final stage in several hundred million years of previous, step-by-step preparation of the blastocyst and the uterine mucosa for such a magnificent event.

—Richard Torpin, MD
(Student of the Human Placenta)
Medical College of Georgia
1931-1974

In its extraembryonic site the primitive streak creates a node-like cell reservoir from which the allantois, a universal caudal appendage of all amniotes and the future umbilical cord of placental mammals emerges. This new insight into the fetal/umbilical relationship may explain the etiology of a large number of umbilical-associated birth defects.

—Karen M. Downs
Department of Anatomy
University of Wisconsin-Madison School of Medicine
NIH *Bioessays*
2009

It has been estimated that 30% of births have some type of umbilical cord finding. This statistic implies a potential for fetal harm that may not be appreciated by scientific and public health authorities. Not knowing how many fetuses are harmed by their umbilical cords prevents research into the issue. If neurological harm can occur as the result of umbilical cord problems, then this mechanism of harm to the fetus needs to be investigated. Every fetus should have the opportunity to begin life with all its God-given talents and abilities. Realistically, this may not be possible, but some physically normal newborns could benefit from a reduction in the risks of a cord mishap. It is estimated that learning disabilities may represent 15% of children today. What if one-third of these learning disabilities are due to some type of cord complication? The issue of cerebral palsy is important, but currently, no solution and few insights exist as to its origin. Preventing the stillbirth of a normal infant would be an important step in identifying cord-related harm. What is the size of the problem, and what best describes each part of the problem of umbilical cord mishaps? Disruption of the umbilical cord supply line is a major source of harm to the developing fetus. It is estimated that every third to fourth delivery has an identifiable umbilical cord abnormality or anomaly. What is unknown is how these findings affect the fetus in degrees. The obvious effect is that stillbirth can result from the closing of the supply line.

The Stillbirth Collaborative Research Network recently reported on the probable or possible cause of death of 512 stillbirths whose mothers consented to complete postmortem examination of their baby. Umbilical cord accidents (UCA) were reported to represent 10% of stillbirths. In Caucasians, the UCA-associated stillbirth rate was 13% and 4% in non-Hispanics and blacks. Nine percent of stillbirths were due to hypertension and 8% due to other maternal medical disorders. A literature review places the UCA-associated stillbirth rate at 15%. These databases do not include stillbirth due to several UCA pathologies such as torsion, multiple cord entanglement, and abnormal placental cord insertion. The main reason for these absences is the belief by some that these abnormalities do not cause actual death or recurrent stillbirth. It is now evident that UCA is more important a cause of stillbirth than pregnancy hypertension or gestational diabetes. It is now necessary to develop protocols to identify and manage this problem.

Recommended Reading

> The Stillbirth Collaborative Research Network Writing Group, Bukowski, R., M. Carpenter, D. Conway, D. Coustan, D. J. Dudley, R. L. Goldenberg, C. J. Hogue, M. A. Koch, C. B. Parker, H. Pinar, U. M. Reddy, G. R. Saade, R. M. Silver, B. J. Stoll, M. W. Varner, M. Willinger. 2011. "Causes of Death Among Stillbirths."
> *JAMA* 306 (22): 2459-2468. doi: 10.1001/jama.2011.1823

The umbilical cord is a multidifferentiated organ. Connection to the placenta is one of its many functions. Located at the lower third of the embryo at the primitive ridge, the proximal portion of the umbilical cord begins to form at the allantoic core domain. Between four and six weeks, as the embryonic disc takes a cylindrical shape, the umbilical cord grows and fuses with the placenta. It elongates away from the placenta, forming umbilical cord vessels and increasing in diameter. There are eight different umbilical cord forms, the genetics of which have yet to be studied. The nature of umbilical cord growth may be determined by paternal genes versus the placental genes. The importance of this is, the umbilical cord is not placental in origin and has its own distinct origins. Scientifically it should be treated as a separate organ of reproduction. The proximal fetal attachment is unique and develops a sac (herniation) by ten weeks. This area houses the guts (intestines) until the twelfth week of gestation. At this time, the umbilical cord is short, usually shorter than the head-to-tail (crown-to-rump) length of the embryo and of proportionately large diameter. It is not able to tolerate rotation about itself or the formed embryo. In fact, as the umbilical cord elongates, the proximal cord encompassing the intestinal pouch cannot be disturbed. The distal initial stalk develops in the center of the placental implantation site. The allantois begins at the pole (end) of the embryo and eventually centers itself in the fetus. By twelve weeks, the intestines leave the proximal cord and return to the stomach, the elongation of the cord begins, and the location of the umbilicus (belly button) positions in the middle third of the embryo. The elongation of the umbilical vein and arteries coincides with the development of Wharton's jelly, an umbilical cord connective tissue, the stem cells of which can used for regeneration of various tissues including the heart.

What umbilical cord fundamental factors might contribute to UCA? Different characteristics in umbilical cord structure and function may predispose a given fetus to UCA under stressful conditions. Umbilical cord properties—tensile strength, diameter, circumference, Wharton's jelly content, weight, and length—may be determined genetically. Umbilical cord development, differentiation, growth, and elongation may depend on the sex of the fetus, its nutrition, and well-being. The anatomical connection of the umbilical cord to the fetus and placenta may be independent issues of growth, development, and separation. The human umbilical cord varies in its microstructure, nerves, and elemental content from arteries to vein. Variations in enzyme content of the cord exist from fetus to placenta. There are umbilical cord-vessel cellular and biochemical differences in the umbilical cords of normal and abnormal fetuses. These differences are also noted in vessel response to temperature between vein and artery. As of 2010, there are very few publications on gene expression of the normal placenta and normal cord. Tissue sampling of the placenta and cord may be location based and not uniform. An examination of umbilical cord tissue in smoking mothers reviewed *mRNA* expression. Validation of three *somatomammotropin* genes showed a high correlation between qPCR and microarray expression, suggesting altered gene expression of the fetus. An examination of umbilical cord tissue in bronchopulmonary dysplasia (BPD) babies showed gene expression of the chromatin remodeling pathway. Aberrations of the attachments can affect the function of the umbilical cord. These differences from fetus to fetus may explain the vulnerability of one fetus over another with a similar UCA (such as nuchal cord and as exampled by the 2009 H1N1 swine flu pandemic, which caused deaths in susceptible patients).

Tensile strength: Several reports have measured the breaking point of the human umbilical cord. Because of the differences among cords in Wharton's jelly, collagen content, and muscle layer structure, there is a range of breakage points and sites. The average load required to break the majority of human umbilical cords is 10-14 lb, the range being 4-24 lb (at term, 1.81-10.89 kg). Cords ruptured 22.5% of the time at the placental end (without description of the attachment). Umbilical cord traction forces of 8 lb usually separated the placenta from the uterus. Otherwise, most cord ruptures were within 12 inches of the fetus. The human umbilical cord is elastic and will stretch to 12.5% of its length. The tensile strength may average 2.5% of fetal weight. As a result, some fetuses may tolerate more traction and loss of slack during entanglement than others. Lastly, *cDNA* microarray analysis of human umbilical vein endothelial cells (HUVECs) under strain point to genetic expression of vasoactive materials and cellular alteration. A condition called mosaicism (more than one pair of genes in the fetus and placenta) has now been reported in the umbilical cord. This suggests that paternal genes may influence cord characteristics more than maternal genes.

Diameter/circumference: The human umbilical cord has a reported average diameter of 1.5 cm and a separately reported average circumference of 3.6 cm after birth. The umbilical vein and artery have been measured before and after birth. The ultrasound average vein diameter is 8 mm with an average artery diameter of 4 mm at term. Various biomechanical characteristics of the umbilical cord such as elasticity, vessel wall thickness, and pressure tolerance have been studied. There is an association with aneuploidy and abnormal diameters.

Umbilical cord cells have a potential to act as multipotential stem cells. These stem cells can transform into anticancer and hematopoietic cells. There may also be potential for anticancer therapy with matrix-derived cells. There are no reported cancers of the umbilical cord.

Length: Cord length can be associated with neurologic abnormalities and fetal positioning Umbilical cord complications increase as the length increases. To understand this correlation, it is important to understand the physiology of the human umbilical cord. Cord length has been frequently measured. One of the largest studies was completed by Pathologist Dr. Richard Naeye. In his book Disorders of the Placenta, Fetus, and Neonate, Dr. Naeye averages the lengths of different umbilical cords at progressively older gestational ages. The cord is believed to elongate until as late as 36 weeks although rapid change occurs until 28 weeks, then slows. The final length of the umbilical cord averages about 61 cm, or 24 inches, according to Percy Malpas, M.D., a British obstetrician who studied cord length in the 1960s. The first pregnancy tends to generate a shorter cord than subsequent pregnancies. Although no published report of a genetic relationship exists for cord length in subsequent pregnancies, there may be one. So why 61 cm? Umbilical cords of whales, porpoises, goats and other mammals are relatively shorter than the human cord. Walker and Rye of Cambridge surmised in the British Medical Journal in 1960 that prehistoric humans evolved length for protection. Nature.s purpose was to allow the mother to pick up the newborn without disturbing the placenta. The event of breast feeding would then separate the placenta - an event which could attract predators. Having the fetus in tow would allow escape for mother and child.

The human umbilical cord can be totally absent or reach a length of 300cm. Research has shown that removal of a key area called the Allantoic Core prior to 6 weeks disrupts cord substance development. Cord vessel development can be disrupted by removing key protiens. Umbilical cord length is the only factor associated and documented as a definite risk factor for poor fetal outcome. There is an association of abnormal cord length with neurological abnormalities and low IQ values. A multivariate analysis of a small sample of pregnancies (n 1087 births) reported an association with long cords and IUGR only. An evaluation of all umbilical cords for extremes of length and development should be considered at all deliveries at this time due to findings in larger studies. There may also be an association with urinary tract abnormalities. There is a tendency for long cords. (>70CM @ 4% of cords) to be familial and repeat in the same mother in subsequent pregnanciesare documented to be directly associated with poor fetal outcome and associated with UCA especially; fetal entanglement, true knots, (sometimes multiple knots) and torsion. Placental changes are associated with long cords suggesting blood flow disruption or increased resistance. Male cords are longer than female cords and term vertex fetuses may have longer lengths than term Breech fetuses (with the duration of presentation unknown). Multigravida cord length may be longer than primagravida cord length (the first pregnancy having a shorter length than the third, this may imply more room for movement-tension or more blood supply/hormone production/ fetal-maternal weight gain). Twin gestations may have fetuses with discordant lengths and shorter lengths than singletons. Short cords (<32cm) was determined in 1910 by a famed Chicago obstetrician, Dr.

Joseph B. DeLee. He reported 32 cm to be the minimal length necessary for a term fetus to deliver. The concept changes, however, when cord insertion site and cord entanglement are considered. This idea is called a relatively short cord. Very short cords less than 20 cm are associated with genetic malformations. When cord lengths were evaluated for IQ, short cords showed a higher incidence of neurologic abnormalities. Today, cord length correlates to several outcomes.. Cords too short and cords too long predispose the fetus to intrauterine dangers. Cord length may also influence fetal position. Umbilical cord function is not readily impaired by longness and venous return from the placenta to the fetus is maintained regardless of length.Torgrim Sørnes, M.D., a Norwegian researcher, observed this. His work suggests that Breech-positioned fetuses have shorter cords due to less activity. This insight suggests that if the fetus persists at remaining Breech, a cord etiology should be considered, and the obstetrician should watch for fetal difficulties during labor. Umbilical cord circumference and diameter are also important measurements. On average, normal umbilical cords are 3.7 cm in circumference with a range of 3 - 5 cm. The diameter range of 1.0 cm to 3.0 cm can suggest an abnormal cord with edema, tumor, or hernia. Dimensions greater than 6 cm circumference should prompt an examination of the cord and fetus. Are shorter cords thicker than longer cords? Although rarely published, it appears that this may be the case. Before cutting any thick cord, it should be checked to ensure that the fetal intestine is not present within the cord. Growth and development of the umbilical cord are dependent upon many factors. Disturbance of these events can lead to fetal compromise or result in fetal compromise. These effects will be described in the next chapter.

Absent or Short (< 35cm) umbilical cords (@ 3% of cords) have been described and reported in cases of congenital anomalies. A short cord may be due to reduced fetal activity (such as with twinning; monoamniotic and conjoined). There is a reported association between fetal movement and bone density. This suggests that decreased fetal movement and short cords and low bone density are related. A primary failure of elongation has been noted in association with Sirenomelia (lack of adequate fetal blood pressure), Shisis, Anencephaly (lack of hypothalamic hormones?), Acardia (cardiac output?) and adhesions (Early Amniotic Rupture Sequence -EARS). There may be additional molecular factors involved in cord lengthening which are not tension related. Genetic origins may also exist and placental imprinted genes may play a role in cord length. These limb-body wall complex (LBWC), although rare, may provide insights into cord development. Placental trisomy 16 is associated with short cord (which may be developmental as a result of restricted fetal movement or directly related to genetic malfunction). Absolutely short cords can interfere with the mechanics of labor and delivery while exhibiting changes in fetal heart rate patterns. This restriction of decent (which is relative to the placental position and insertion) leads to an increase in the incidence of cesarean section, forcep and vacuum extractions. Relatively short cords (lengths compromised by fetal entanglement causing loss of slack) can interfere with delivery as well. As of 2010, there is no published report of a short cord recurrence or familial genetic inheritance. There is one report of prenatal diagnosis of a short cord.

RECOMMENDED READING

Study of length of Umbilical Cord and Fetal Outcome; A study of 1000 deliveries. Balkawade U.N., Shinde M.A. J Obstet Gynecol India 2012;65(5) 520-25.

Long umbilical cords: long umbilical cords (> 70 cm at 4% of cords) are documented to be directly associated with poor fetal outcome and associated with UCA, especially fetal entanglement, true knots (sometimes multiple), and torsion. Placental changes are associated with long cords, suggesting blood flow disruption or increased resistance. Male cords are longer than female cords, and term vertex fetuses may have longer lengths than term breech fetuses (with the duration of presentation unknown). Multigravida cord length may be longer than primigravida cord length (the first pregnancy having a shorter length than the third, this may imply more room for movement-tension or more blood supply/hormone production/fetal and maternal weight gain). Twin gestations may have fetuses with discordant lengths and shorter lengths than singletons. Single umbilical artery-vessel structure is increased in long cords. There are no studies considering maternal smoking, alcohol, caffeine, or cocaine ingestion and umbilical cord length in humans (animal studies report shorter cord lengths than controls). Umbilical cord function is not readily impaired by length, and venous return from the placenta to the fetus is maintained regardless of length. There may be an association between viscoelastic behavior of the cord and protection against excessive elongation (which means fetal movement may have a limited effect on cord elongation). There are no studies measuring the umbilical cord prenatally with ultrasound and evaluating the risk factor of cord length for poor fetal outcomes.

Umbilical cord-vessel number: Reports of five vessels, four vessels, fused cords in twins, and two-vessel cords have associated fetal conditions. The best one studied of these findings is umbilical cords with one artery and one vein, single umbilical artery (SUA).

Single umbilical artery (SUA) cases have been reported with a variety of genetic, anomalous, and stillbirth outcomes. There are SUA findings associated with trisomy malformations but no confirmed genetic sequence associations with UCA to date. SUA is considered to be a developmental UCA associated with disturbance of fetal blood flow. There are two forms of SUA: a helical form and a straight form. Many observations have been published about this umbilical cord maldevelopment that is seen at 7% of abortus up to twenty-eight weeks, at 7% twins, and occurs at 1% of term pregnancies. There may be an association between the left or right umbilical artery that is absent and increased risk of fetal abnormalities. There may be several categories of SUA depending on which vessel represents the umbilical artery (vitelline, allantoic, R or L umbilical). There is also a difference in malformations depending on whether the right or left vein persists. SUA is associated with stillbirth with an incidence of 3%-20%. SUA is common in twins and diabetic pregnancies, in association with long cords and small placentas. Finding an SUA on ultrasound screening should place the pregnancy on alert for associated developments. Trisomies, especially those with mosaic genetics, should be reviewed for fetal anomalies. A finding of SUA entanglement or decreased fetal weight should prompt closer fetal evaluation.

Recommended Reading

Isolated single umbilical artery and fetal karyotype.

Dagklis T[1], Defigueiredo D, Staboulidou I, Casagrandi D, Nicolaides KH. Ultrasound Obstet Gynecol. 2010 Sep;36(3):291-5.

Umbilical cord-vessel morphology may be a risk factor for the fetus. The normal umbilical cord may have been best illustrated and described in 1882 by E. S. Tarnier: an arterial pair mildly helical around a straight vein (with helical muscle bundles by microscopy). Umbilical cord morphology (design) is established by ten to twelve weeks. The normal umbilical cord has six to eight embedded helixes. These helixes do not unwind, are 360 degrees, and cannot be untwisted. The term *helixes* is the proper nomenclature (not *coils, curls, turns, spirals, chirals,* or *twists*).Umbilical cord helixes are fundamental to umbilical cord development and normal function. Other morphologies should be considered abnormal. There are differences in umbilical cord shape that may predispose the fetus to UCA. There may be eight different types (forms) of umbilical cords. There are biochemical differences within the umbilical cord from placenta to fetus that are distinct in compromised fetuses versus normal fetuses. It is theorized that several factors may determine umbilical cord shape. Fetal cardiac output, predominance of umbilical artery blood flow, and fetal symmetry may be important. Study by Doppler velocimetry of cord length, artery pairs, and helical types have suggested some differences that may be important, but fetal outcomes were not always reported. There may be an inherent role of the umbilical cord to assist the fetal heart. If so, umbilical cord morphology may change this assist action or "pulsometer." Thrombosis of the umbilical vein may disrupt this pump-assist action and lead to stillbirth. Previous studies on UCA have not fully considered the differences that may be inherent in these different forms.

Umbilical cord attachments: There is specialized anatomy for the umbilical cord attachment to the placenta and fetus. Failure of these attachments will cause fetal death. The umbilical ring is designed to allow for fetal growth without umbilical cord detachment until delivery. The umbilical ring is innervated, and these nerves have branches that connect to the vagus trunks and phrenic nerves. There are connecting branches to the right adrenal gland and maybe to the proximal umbilical cord. This neuronal pattern may suggest an umbilical ring to the ductus venosus feedback system, which partly regulates blood flow to the fetal cardiovascular system. Failure of proper umbilical cord development at the fetal attachment can cause stillbirth. As stated previously, absent umbilical cord syndrome is fatal. Other defects can be due to embryonic structures and remnants at the proximal cord. Proximal umbilical cysts, urachal anomalies, and vitelline-vessel anomalies have been well described in pathology texts. Periumbilical skin length may also have extremes, of which long skin lengths have been noted in dysmorphic children and UCA in horses. Velamentous insertion (VI) comes in various forms. It is an abnormal attachment to the membranes instead of the placenta. Its impact on the fetus is dependent on placental position (360 degrees in the uterus and insertion direction dependent). Velamentous insertion over the uterine cervix is called vasa previa. It is now possible to identify VI by multiple methods: ultrasound, color Doppler, 3-D imaging, which includes MRI. The prenatal diagnosis of VI is now a requirement of twenty-first-century obstetrical practice. Once diagnosed, this UCA can be managed, and stillbirth can be prevented. VI can be visualized by the eighteen-week to twenty-week ultrasound.

Recommended Reading

Risk Factors and Outcomes of Velamentous and Marginal Cord Insertions; A population-based study of 634,741 pregnancies: Cebbing, T Kiserud, S Johnson, S Albrichtsen PLOS; July 2013 Volume 8

The responsibilities of the cord are numerous. For example, the cord manages its own growth, elongation, and expansion; accommodates increasing blood flow; and possibly assists the fetal heart. It also must regulate blood flow and its fluidity (thickness/thinness). In addition, the umbilical arteries and vein contain muscular coats that allow constriction of the vessels at birth or dilation of the vessels during growth. The umbilical cord also must produce its own chemistry to prepare for its role in birth and separation from the newborn umbilicus (a process which takes seven to ten days). Located within the cord are the umbilical vein and arteries. The relationship of the umbilical vein to the umbilical arteries changes with development. These changes can result in cord abnormalities, which will be discussed in the next chapter. Initially, two arteries send blood with waste products from the embryo to the afterbirth (placenta), and the one umbilical vein sends oxygen and nutrient-enriched blood to the embryo from the placenta. This circulation pattern must respond over time to the constantly changing fetal requirements and demands.

Rare developmental changes, which can occur to the embryonic umbilical cord, are persistent of the right vitelline vein, creating a four-vessel cord with two arteries and two veins. The reverse of this is obliteration of an artery and vein and the development of a two-vessel cord with one artery and one vein. There also exists a description of a double cord within separate vessel duplication. Genetic problems are seen with two-vessel cords where fetuses with multiple malformations have defective organs that are not compatible with life. Maldevelopment of the genitourinary system such as bladder and kidney has been noticed. Although these relationships are known, obstetrics currently does not place any added concern on pregnancies with two-vessel cords. No remedy for these anomalies presently exists. Umbilical cord vessels may multiply and branch under stressful conditions. For example, heavy smoking is associated with multiple channels in the umbilical cord. Hypoxia (the decrease of available oxygen) has been determined as the stimulus for opening of early vestigial vessels of the cord, once closed at ten weeks. These findings of rechanneled embryonic vessels are also associated with fetal compromise and stillbirths. A trend was also noted in which first-time pregnancies had more vascular branching than multiple-birth mothers. Research indicates a 2% probability of this cord finding. How the umbilical cord elongates and grows is unknown. As it grows, it changes the relationship between the vein and arteries. These changes may or may not predispose the growing fetus to blood flow disturbances or mechanical disturbances between the fetus and umbilical cord. The umbilical cord is traditionally thought to stretch or elongate depending on the activity of the fetus. Active fetuses are believed to have longer cords on the whole than less active fetuses. Twins and triplets, because of restricted movement, have been shown to have cords, on the average, shorter than their single counterparts. Boys have longer cords than girls. Nonidentical twins have varying cord lengths when compared to each other. Nonidentical twin A can have a cord twice the length of twin B. Also, twins A and B can have different cord architectures where one is straight and one is helical.

Rare instances exist in which no cord develops at all, the fetus being attached directly to the placenta at the umbilicus. Other reports in Chinese and French literature cite cords as long as 300 cm in length. The umbilical cord appears to have organ-like properties. These properties are prone to disturbance under certain conditions that can affect the fetus. Just as a heart can fail pumping or the liver and kidney can fail filtering the body's chemistry and waste products, the umbilical cord can fail in its role of being a supply line.

Wharton's Jelly

Wharton's jelly is a specialized tissue serving many purposes for the developing fetus. Its specialized cells contain gelatin-like mucus that encases fibers. These properties give it an elastic and cushiony effect, which can tolerate the vibration, bending, stretching, and twisting of an active fetus. In addition, it holds the vessels together, may regulate blood flow, plays a role in providing nutrition to the fetus, stores chemistry for the onset of labor, and protects the supply line. Umbilical cords without much Wharton's jelly are more prone to compression, and complete absence is usually associated with fetal death. If an umbilical cord is twisted or knotted, it is more likely to tighten where there is less resistance, such as an area low in Wharton's jelly. It is believed that males have more Wharton's jelly content than do females and that good nutrition increases the amount. Wharton's jelly tends to reduce with gestational age and can disappear when pregnancies go beyond forty weeks. Because these cases tend to have fetal heart rate changes, the level of Wharton's jelly is a consideration when obstetricians plan the deliveries of pregnancies low on amniotic fluid.

Umbilical Cord Design

How the umbilical cord is built has long been of interest to anatomists. A look at all mammals shows a variety of design adaptations. In humans, it has been determined that there are several designs. What these differences mean to the fetus is unknown. Attempts by several noted scientists to understand how the umbilical cord works have taught us that the cord is more like an organ rather than a rigid conduit (pipeline).

Not all cords are alike. Just as there are different kinds of hair (curly/straight, thick/thin), there are different kinds of cords. Most cords (99%) have three vessels although some (1%) have only two, and even less have four. The relationship between the normal vein and two arteries is usually parallel (figure 7). This parallel configuration can vary, however, and may imply effects that can alter blood supply to the fetus. Variances include arteries that are together or separated with each artery lateral to the vein (figure 8). Another variance is arteries that wind around the vein while the vein remains central in the cord. This is sometimes referred to as spiraled arteries, but *helical* is the preferred term (figure 9). The vein can also parallel the arteries in a helical configuration, and the vein can wind around the arteries. Several researchers have concentrated on these differences and suggest that umbilical cords of absolutely straight designs may be more prone to disruptions of blood flow. If these observations are verified, it may be important to know the cord design prior to delivery. The location of umbilical cord attachment to the fetus and placenta is also important. Placental attachments can be in the center, off-center, on the edge, or in the membranes. Membranous insertions of the umbilical cord are called velamentous insertions. These placental cord designs have flaws that can lead to cord tears. Currently, little research has been done to develop prenatal diagnostic criteria. Umbilical attachment of the cord can vary and predispose the infant to hernias at the umbilicus and constriction of the cord. Although these are uncommon findings, future research will allow a more accurate evaluation of the umbilicus. Amniotic bands can interfere with both ends of the umbilical cord. For example, the amniotic membrane can leave remnants in the form of fibrous bands, which can stiffen and occlude the blood circulation through the cord.

These events are reproductive mishaps that have no current remedy. In order to begin the process of creating solutions to umbilical cord-related complications, understanding cord function and design must be thorough.

Umbilical Cord Abnormalities and Anomalies

Throughout human history, stillbirths have been associated with umbilical cord findings. These findings vary, and some are more common than others.

Scientifically, umbilical cord changes and effects are described several ways. To start, the umbilical cord can develop design flaws that can lead to fetal harm. These flaws are called umbilical cord abnormalities:

Table 1	
Short Cords	less than 35 cm
Long Cords	more than 70 cm
Two-Vessel Cords	one artery/one vein
Four-Vessel Cords	two arteries/two veins
Velamentous Insertions	inserted on the membranes
Marginal Insertions	inserted on the placental edge
Constriction of the Umbilicus	lack of Wharton's jelly at the fetal insertion
Wharton's jelly cysts	mucinous Myxoid Edema Growths and Cysts of the Umbilical Cord Umbilical Artery Angioma/Aneurysm Umbilical Vein Varices/ False Knots Hematoma/Teratoma/Thrombosis/Rupture

These abnormal umbilical cords are predisposed to rupture, mechanical failure, entanglement, disruption of labor, uterine malfunction, and premature labor. The ultimate effects are disturbance of the lifeline and derangement of blood flow to the fetus. The difficulty lies in the fact that these abnormalities are silent and invisible. Short umbilical cords (less than 35 cm) are predisposed to rupture and prevention of fetal descent during labor. Very short cords, less than 25 cm, are associated with genetic malformations. Short umbilical cords need to be considered relative to their attachments to the placenta. The further the attachment is from the cervix, the less likely the fetus can be born vaginally, requiring a C-section. In addition, fetal heart rate changes will be more likely to occur during monitoring, creating concern for all involved in the labor process. Very short umbilical cords, less than 25 cm, have been associated with neurologic disorders, IQs less than 80, and cerebral palsy. There is an increase in stillbirth risk with short and relatively short cords. This risk may be as much as six times more likely, especially when other factors like toxemia are involved. Short cords and cigarette smoking tend to result in small babies, called IUGR (intrauterine growth retarded). It is difficult to unravel the relationships mentioned above since some fetuses may incur neurologic damage, which predisposes them to decreased activity and leads to decreased cord length. Long umbilical cords (longer than 70 cm) are associated with a number of circumstances that can impact fetal life. Leonardo da Vinci studied cord length and believed it was a proportional/natural relationship of 1 to 1 (cord length = fetal age in weeks). Although this is not precisely correct, da Vinci was correct in that it is proportional. Biological and physical principles that dictate the shape of a starfish, tree leaf, or nautilus shell determine the positive or negative relationship between the fetus and its umbilical cord (and probably placenta). Fetal activity is believed to determine umbilical cord growth. This mechanical stimulus may be a direct or indirect factor. How does the umbilical cord grow and elongate? Biochemical and cellular mechanisms must be at work. All these molecular genetic pieces are potentially at risk for failure by inside or outside disturbances. Growth factors have been identified in the umbilical cord. In addition, studies in twins suggest a genetic control or modulation of length. Length can also be influenced by amniotic fluid volume and anything that constricts fetal movement. Umbilical cords are also innervated to a degree near the umbilicus. The role this plays or whether there is an influence on cord development is currently unknown. Of all those multiple variables influencing cord length, the most important variable needs to be determined. It is unknown whether individual cell enlargement or cell division and multiplication cause cord growth. Many different cells such as muscle cells, endothelial cells, fibroblasts, connective cells, and amniotic cells must all do the same thing. Insight into this aspect of fetal development may help understand anomalies of the cord. Microscopic comparison of long and short cords may reveal differences of structure. Thickness or thinness of vessel walls, composition of Wharton's jelly, and artery-vein interrelationships may be important findings that explain long-cord susceptibility to various events. Two-vessel cords occur in about 1% of births. The connection to fetal harm or well-being is unclear. These umbilical cords have one artery and one vein. The dominant artery origination (left or right inside the fetus) determines whether or not congenital malformations may be present. It is accepted that these cords may predispose the fetus to stillbirth compared to a normal three-vessel cord. The risk of stillbirth can be six times greater than normal, especially when other factors such as toxemia exist. Whether or not other variables are involved remains to be determined. Development of a single umbilical artery cord may be associated with maternal smoking, drug exposure, placental abnormalities, and maternal diabetes. Whether or not all infants with a two-vessel cord are predisposed to some difficulty remains to be seen. The mechanism of how one artery is obliterated versus undeveloped may be important to understanding this issue. Four-vessel umbilical cords are rare and are mentioned to emphasize the vulnerability of cord vessels to malformation. Not all umbilical cords are alike, and nonidentical twins can have nonidentical cords. Proper development of the embryo and its supply line is an important step toward a healthy fetus and newborn. Maldevelopment of the supply line from the start can predispose the fetus to harm. Another important step in umbilical cord development is the connection of the fetus and placenta to each other. The fetal connection is specialized and has a specific architecture. This design needs to function as a secure tether for the fetus, as a disrupter for umbilical separation (in mammals, the cord tears free or is chewed free), and perhaps, as a sensor for blood flow into the fetus, and must merge with the skin. Researchers have identified nerve endings near the umbilical insertion of the cord in the

Wharton's jelly. These end nests may play a role in communicating with fetal valves, called shunts, relative to blood volume-wave properties entering the fetal circulation through the umbilical vein at the level of the liver and heart. When the umbilical end is malformed, constriction or coarctation occurs, stopping blood flow. How this happens is unknown. At the other end of the supply line, the fetal arteries enter the placenta with a membranous support tether and distribute in a branching manner. When the placenta develops, it sometimes migrates and dissolves from its original site. This sometimes can result in what appears to be a relocation of the placenta. The placenta tissue dissolves, leaving a membrane (the amnion), which can then be the connection (insertion) site of the umbilical cord. This results in the umbilical cord placental end looking like it is connected to the edge of the placenta (called a marginal or battledore insertion) and a membranous insertion called a (velamentous) insertion. Another variation is called a furcate cord insertion in which the cord does not connect to the placenta, but its branching elements do; however, no membranous insertion exists. These malformations account for another 0.5% to 1% of all births and are observed to increase in premature labor, premature birth, fetal stillbirth, and neurologic harm.

The risk of cord-vessel rupture is increased with an abnormal cord insertion. The difficulty of managing an incident such as cord rupture is great. What makes the mystery even more complicated is the location of the cord insertion in the uterus. If the membranous insertion is over the cervical opening, the risk of tearing and fetal blood loss is great. If a marginal insertion is against the sacrum (lower backbone), the risk of compression and fetal circulation disruption is great as the fetus descends into the pelvis. This relationship of vessel location to fetal location has caused sudden fetal distress and the need to activate a surgical team for an emergency C-section. It is unknown how often this happens during day-to-day obstetrical care as the attention is on the fetus, not the placenta, its location, or its cord-insertion architecture. Umbilical cords may have eight different types of design. The extremes are very helical cords (95%) and completely straight cords (5%). The association between umbilical vein and arteries can vary where veins wind around arteries, veins and arteries are parallel, and arteries wind around veins. The veins can be parallel with the arteries as well (10%).

Very helical designs (spiraled, coiled, and curled) may predispose the fetus to certain blood flow changes, and very straight designs may be susceptible to compression. It is unknown what the fetal effects are, but some evidence points to supply-line vulnerability when the design is faulty. Add to this other variables such as placental location and umbilical cord insertion site and the combination becomes a significant factor in determining the well-being of the fetus. Knowing these details may provide important insights into the development of fetal harm. Wharton's jelly, although apparently inert looking, may be an important chemical factory for the fetus. Additionally, its components and cellular makeup can predispose the fetus to the formation of tumors, cysts, and edema. Edema is not an infrequent finding at delivery of a newborn (10%). It is usually limited to small sections of the umbilical cord and associated with trauma due to fetal behavior. Extensive involvement of the cord is associated with complications of pregnancy such as toxemia and infections. When cause is due to fetal circulatory disturbances, fetal heart failure may predispose the cord to edema, which is associated with an increased risk of stillbirth. Tumors can develop in Wharton's jelly. Although rare, teratomas have been reported. Teratomas grow to large sizes and can disrupt vessels and blood flow. Embryonic features of the umbilical cord can produce six types of remnants, some of which look like hemangiomas, blood vessels which, together, look like small varicose veins in a bundle. Other structures such as vitelline duct remnants and urachal duct remnants can be seen. Those changes are very infrequent but should be considered if an enlargement or localized mass is seen in the cord. Hematomas (bleeds into the substance of the cord) can occur and mimic these rare tumors. The possible association with fetal defects must always be considered. As the fetus ages, it is believed that Wharton's jelly recedes. This becomes an important issue when deciding to deliver a postdate infant, where the due date has been passed without delivery. Loss of Wharton's jelly may put the fetus at risk of cord compression and, therefore, fetal harm.

Growths and Swellings of Umbilical Cord Vessels

Like any vessel in the human adult body, umbilical cord vessels can develop sacs, protrusions, bulges, and varicosities. For example, cord vessels can protrude and thrombose like varicose veins or hemorrhoidal veins. In addition, the umbilical vein sometimes bunches up on itself, creating the appearance of a false knot or of multiple varicosities; these spaces can act like quiet pools of blood that can clot and predispose the fetus to a thromboembolism. The clot can break free and enter the fetal circulation or can obstruct cord blood flow. The umbilical arteries can develop similar pockets called aneurysms. These bulges in the arterial vessel wall can rupture and lead to fetal hemorrhages in the uterus. These alterations of structure can predispose the cord to rupture as well. Human umbilical arteries consist of two layers of muscle fibers, the outer layer being three-fourths of the wall thickness and an inner layer. The design of the muscle cells is parallel, where the inner layer runs with the vessel lengthwise and the outer layer surrounds the vessel like a spiral staircase. A thin layer of cells lines the vessel opening, and an outer layer is formed by connective tissue and Wharton's jelly. This architecture allows constriction and shortening of the vessel. Defects in this structure can occur that may predispose the umbilical arteries to failure. A type of architectural defect is called umbilical cord-vessel segmental thinning. In this malformation (1%), umbilical vessel walls are missing a layer of muscle, therefore weakening the vessel. Related observations include fetal anomalies and perinatal problems. These fetuses are predisposed to stillbirth, meconium, and fetal heart rate decelerations. All in all, when a combination of defects results, the risk of umbilical cord failure begins to become important. It is unknown how many placentas and umbilical cords contain a variety of architectural anomalies or abnormalities that lead to miscarriage. It is unknown how much fetal harm may be the result of faulty placentation and cord alterations, such as straight cord segments resulting from the molding of Wharton's jelly due to long-term compression of an entangled cord.

Future research into these issues will be both exciting and fruitful. The integration of the anatomy (structure), biochemistry (substance), and physiology (function) of the umbilical cord will allow the emergence of a new awareness of three structures to manage in pregnancy: the placenta, umbilical cord, and fetal unit.

How the Human Umbilical Cord Works (Physiology)

What is remarkable about the umbilical cord is that it is a blood vessel without branches. This is unique compared to the large blood vessels of the adult body—the aorta and vena cava. Its properties, therefore, are different in some respects and alike in others. The umbilical cord has two-way traffic: the arteries carry blood pumped by the heart away from the fetus, and this circulation surrounds the vein normally; the umbilical vein returns blood to the fetus from the placenta rejuvenated with oxygen and nutrients and devoid of waste products. How this happens is still surrounded by mystery. The fetal heart cannot expand or work harder because it is surrounded by a fluid-filled lung, like pushing against a water bed. Therefore, as the fetus steadily grows exponentially and three-dimensionally, how does it accommodate the increased blood volume it needs over time? As the fetus grows, the cord elongates and grows in diameter. The fetus has to work against a larger column of fluid and tissue resistance at the placental end. It has been estimated that by thirty-one weeks, the umbilical cord must carry seventy quarts of blood per day, moving at four miles an hour. This remarkable organ also must participate in fetal growth milestones; additionally, it may act as an assist pump to the fetal heart. This assist pump may be designed to help the fetus over difficult growth proportions that may exist at twenty weeks, twenty-four weeks, twenty-eight weeks, and thirty-two weeks—times that are known for premature labor to appear. The extra stress on the fetus may require that the cord be designed correctly so that it can have properties of an assist mechanism or pump. This theory, proposed in the 1950s, requires that the arteries surround the vein in the proper architecture. If this is so, then future research into this issue may explain fetal effects secondary to cord design. To date, no assist-pump property has been detected in the umbilical cord. How blood flow is regulated in addition to being carried by the umbilical cord is unclear.

Cord length does not significantly affect blood flow dynamics; however, blood flow must meet some resistance for the circulation to work. As a result, the umbilical arteries are surrounded with four layers of smooth muscle to maintain a certain amount of muscular tone. The umbilical vein is not as muscled. The system operates fully dilated, but stimuli from chemistry or hormones can affect the system and cause constriction.

This must happen at birth to reduce blood loss. In larger mammals, the cord must constrict from the placenta to the fetus for the fetus to avoid anemia. In the human, similar mechanisms may be available chemically. Regulation of blood flow, vessel constriction at birth, and blood-loss prevention may be the roles of these vessel-active substances. Some of these substances originate in the placenta. Researchers using ultrasonography recently have been able to measure umbilical blood flow with color Doppler imaging. This technique allows visualization of the blood vessels based on the movement of the blood itself. These studies also suggest that the umbilical vein, arteries, and placenta act as assist pumps of sorts to the fetal heart. Measurement of blood flow allows the obstetrician to determine whether enough blood volume is circulating in the placenta to provide nutrition and oxygen to the fetus. Under certain conditions, this blood flow can be reduced and circulation in the placenta altered to create a growth-affected fetus, intrauterine growth retardation (IUGR). In essence, it is a way of determining the fetus's blood pressure. These findings become important because, in addition to the potential for fetal harm or stillbirth, important lifetime tendencies are emerging. The fetus seems to have the ability to set its vital signs for its adult life. If stressed, the IUGR fetus sets blood pressure and heart function, which can predispose the fetus to adult heart attack. These mechanisms are just beginning to be understood, and the umbilical cord may be an important part of the mystery.

A case of a term stillbirth with a straight umbilical cord design with an abnormal placenta, a marginal umbilical cord insertion, and a double nuchal cord was reported from Paris, France, in 1893.

Table II — Umbilical Cord Morphology

VESSEL NUMBER	VESSEL PATTERN	VESSEL FORM
Five Vessels	< .01% V/A$_4$	
Four Vessels	< .1% V/A$_3$, V$_2$/A$_2$	
Three Vessels	85% Straight Vein V$_S$/A$_H$	
	V$_S$/A$_H$ Paired	
	V$_S$/A$_H$ Even	
	5%-8% Straight Vein V$_S$/A$_S$ V$_S$/A$_S$/Pair	
	@>1% Helical Vein Straight Arteries	
	@<1% Helical Vein Helical Arteries V$_H$/A$_H$	
Two Vessels	1%-2% Straight Vein Straight Artery V$_S$/A$_S$ V$_S$/A$_H$	

* V$_S$ - Vein Straight, V$_H$ - Vein Helical, A$_H$ - Artery Helical, A$_S$ - Artery Straight

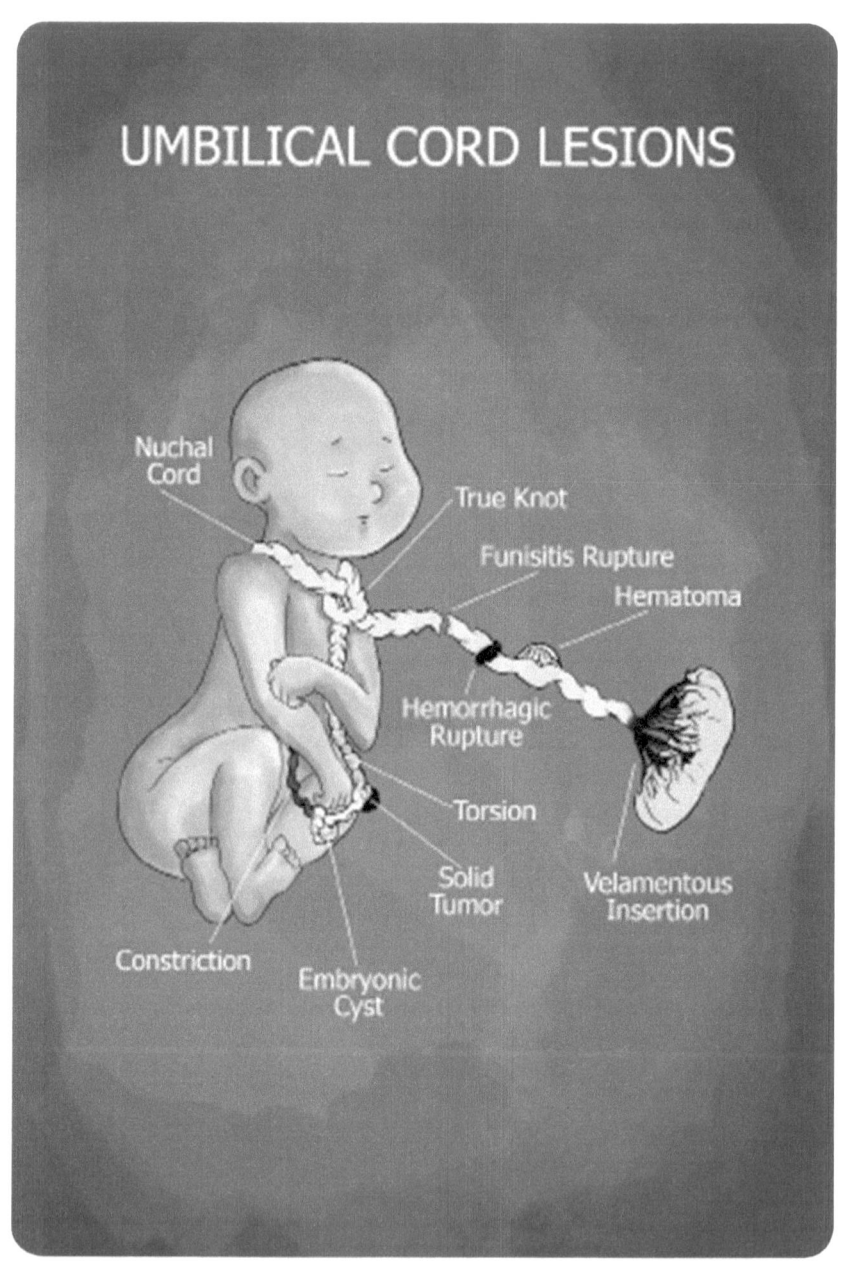

Heifetz, S. A. "Pathology of the umbilical cord." *Pathology of the Placenta*. 2nd edition. Edited by S. H. Lewis and E. Perrin. NY, NY: Churchill Livingstone.

CHAPTER TWO

The Umbilical Cord: The Problems of Supply and Demand

For the layman and more so to the obstetrician, [the umbilical cord] presents a potential hazard during delivery. It is highly desirable that umbilical cords should be examined at delivery.
—Bholanath B. Nadkarni
Professor of Pathology
University of Ottawa/Ontario
Canada, 1969

Many pathologic features of the umbilical cord affect fetal well-being adversely.
—Kurt Benirschke, MD
Professor Emeritus
Department of Pathology University Medical Center
San Diego, California, 1994

Disruption of the umbilical cord (the fetal supply line) may be a source of harm to the developing fetus. An estimated 30% of pregnancies carried to term have some type of umbilical placental abnormality. This means that every third to fourth delivery has an identifiable umbilical cord abnormality or anomaly. What is unknown is how these findings affect the fetus and to what degree. This chapter discusses the types of umbilical cords and their potential inherent complications. The obvious unwanted effect of supply-line disruption is stillbirth. The most dramatic example of this obstruction is an emergency called prolapsed umbilical cord. Prolapse of the cord occurs when a fetus is not properly positioned in the pelvis. Membranes rupture and wash the cord out of the cervix in front of the fetal buttock or head. When the fetal body engages the cervix, the cord is compressed, and blood flow to the fetus ceases. If the patient has the good fortune of being near an operating room, the fetus has ten minutes before harm begins. If a C-section can be performed quickly enough, the infant usually survives without harm. Many variations of this event exist in which factors such as time, degree of compression, and age of the fetus play a role. Yet the common thread among these variations is immediate danger to the fetus. Compression of the umbilical cord obstructs blood flow to and from the fetus. This total obstruction denies the fetus oxygen and blood flow pressure, and it releases stress factors from endocrine organs that contribute to fetal harm.

Umbilical cord compression clearly plays a role in disturbing the well-being of the fetus. The effects of incomplete cord compression are unknown. These impacts are altered by different effects at different gestational ages under various conditions at varying intervals. Current obstetrics continues to debate these issues. Although stillbirth clearly can be caused by a variety of mechanisms creating cord compression, prolapse of the umbilical cord is the only witnessed event that is acknowledged and accepted as a fatal cause-effect complication. The chance of having a prolapsed cord at birth is 1 out of 239 cases to 1 out of 865 cases. The reported chance of fetal loss from a prolapsed cord is 8.6% to 49% of these prolapse occurrences. Similar mechanisms can occur inside the uterus with the same results. One such occurrence is that it can take place with monoamniotic twins. These twins have no barrier between them and can entangle their cords. Stillbirths often occur in one twin or both because of knots and encirclement. It is accepted that these mechanisms do cause stillbirth. On the basis of this knowledge, examination and anticipation of other cord complications are not difficult (table 1). Obstetrical thought now accepts that monoamniotic twins can interfere with each other's umbilical cord. Pregnancies of monoamniotic twins showing no other risk factors or complications are monitored carefully for this supply-line disruption. Published case reports have been described of entangled twins with multiple knots. Intensive surveillance was needed for these monoamniotic twins. These reports have described early intervention when fetal heart rate changes suggested the need for delivery as early as thirty-one weeks. If this concept is recognized for monoamniotic twins, why is it not recognized for single fetuses with cord anomalies or abnormalities?

Worldwide frequency (incidence) of umbilical cord events and stillbirths (mortality)
To date, a world literature review suggests the following:
U C A Incidence Mortality
Single umbilical artery .2%-3.6% 7%
Non-coiled cords 4.3% Unknown
True Knots 1% 6%
Nuchal Cords 14%-30% Unknown
Body Loops 1% 10%
Short Cords Unknown Unknown
Velamentous Cords .54%-2%, 17% 30%

Regardless of mechanisms such as prolapsed cord or twins, the pathophysiology is the same: supply line deprivation, restriction of blood flow, and reduction of oxygen and nutrients to the fetus to the degree that injury or death can occur. What does such a mechanism look like? Again, 30% of fetuses delivered have some finding. What are the varied types of cord abnormalities and accidents that can affect the fetus? Some observations from history give us clues. Leonardo da Vinci was not only an artist but also a sculptor and engineer. He recognized in the human form the same principles of proportion as seen in nature. The Greeks had defined many proportions and believed them keys to understanding life. The fetus is proportioned to itself. The early fetus is seen in thirds and the growing fetus in fourths. The term fetus can be seen in fifths, and it can develop entanglement once the umbilical cord is proportionally long. This seems to suggest the point at which the cord begins to pose a danger. This point begins with the cord being four-fifths as long as the fetal head-to-toe length. At this length, the neck can be encircled 360 degrees. This can often happen after ten to twelve weeks' gestational age. A cord of lesser proportional length can't completely encircle the neck. Cord length plays a role in how a fetus develops, how labor is tolerated, and how delivery occurs. What are the different cord-length effects that have been reported in the medical literature?

Absent umbilical cords: If the umbilical cord does not develop, the fetus can develop but can be malformed. The fetus is directly attached to the placenta at the abdomen and usually develops defects. Fetuses without cords have been born by C-section. Without an umbilical cord, life is usually not possible. Yet this concept was not always apparent. The roles played by the placenta, cord, and fetal heart were not realized until the late 1700s.

Short umbilical cords: A cord can be short (20 cm) but can allow delivery if it is attached to the placenta near the cervix. Yet, as previously described, short umbilical cords can affect the fetus. Restriction of movement may occur for genetic or other reasons. Fetal movements may predispose the cord to compression, constriction, and during labor, failure to progress through the birth canal. Short cords can also be responsible for fetal distress during labor, separation of the placenta, and rupture of the umbilical cord prenatally or during labor. In addition, short cords can predispose the umbilical vein and arteries to tears, which can lead to hematomas (vessel rupture) of the cord. Inversion of the uterus (inside out and a medical emergency) can occur from traction on a short cord. Dr. Smellie describes a case of this type. A relatively short cord is a cord that is entangled with the fetus. Although the length is normal, it is caught over the shoulder or around the arm or neck and uses up slack, becoming mechanically unable to allow vaginal delivery. Disruption, compression, and rupture of the cord can occur in a cord that is relatively short. Prenatally addressing a condition of this type will be discussed in chapter 5.

Long umbilical cords: As previously described, a long cord would be considered greater than 70 cm although 90 cm has been used as the measurement. Perhaps a long cord in an abnormal sense should be defined as the length of cord that can cause fetal harm by entanglement.

If so, such a cord would be four-fifths as long as the fetus. Long cords become a problem when circumstances predispose the cord to prolapse (slip out of the womb) and are more likely to prolapse simply because there is more of it. In addition, the umbilical cord is heavier than amniotic fluid and therefore sinks. When visualizing the cord with ultrasound, a cord may seem suspended in the amniotic fluid because of hydrostatic pressure and position. It may appear to float at the top of the uterus, depending on the mother's position. Some papers even comment that the cord floats. Yet the cord does not float; it sinks. The cord can find its way toward the cervix. It always falls away from the fetus even if the fetus chooses to handle it. This sinking property of the cord may be important in preventing cord entanglement. It may be nature's way of reducing the risk of the fetus harming itself. The cord usually bunches up in front of the fetus, commonly near its legs and feet. Long cords may make themselves more available to the fetus and enable the fetus to mouth the cord like a pacifier or handle the cord like a toy. Whether or not this is preferable depends on whether cord blockage is present during the sucking and handling. These simple fetal behaviors may play an important role in fetal well-being and development. Reflexes may exist that serve the purpose of short-duration cord play.

How hard a fetus can squeeze its fist at a given gestational age is unknown. Knowing whether the fetus can grab the umbilical cord and obstruct its own blood flow would be helpful. The grasp would have to exceed its own blood pressure and squeeze with a pressure greater than the fetal systolic pressure (60 mm Hg). Could the strength of some fetuses be a disadvantage? Could the thickness or thinness of cords predispose the cord blood flow to collapse if squeezed? Does the fetus faint and let go? Some anecdotal reports suggest that all these scenarios are possible. A long cord in and of itself is not dangerous. What becomes dangerous is the way in which the fetus interacts with its supply line. The Collaborative Project, a national study of over fifty-five thousand pregnancies, concluded that long cords are associated with fetal entanglement. The key here is to understand that entanglement depends on fetal repositioning in the uterus. Does the umbilical cord itself cause the problem, or does the fetus have to cause the problem? What does the fetus do to become entangled? Are there identifiable factors contributing to an active fetus (one which frequently repositions itself in the uterus and increases its chance of cord entanglement)? Lastly, what role does the mother play when she is active, and does diet play a role? Dietary factors and fetal behavior are currently being investigated. Maternal exercise is also being studied relative to its effect on the fetus. Fetal behavior over time is an active area of research. Scientists are looking for patterns that could mean the difference between well-being and illness.

> A better understanding of the physiology of pregnancy and labor has done away with the theories that the activity of the mother causes coiling of the cord. (Gardiner 1922)

Nuchal Cords: When a fetus's umbilical cord crosses itself 360 degrees around the neck, it has a nuchal cord. Dr. J. Selwyn Crawford of the British Medical Research Council first defined this problem in 1962 as the condition in which the umbilical cord is wound at least once around the neck of the fetus. This initial description was applied to a study that made the following conclusion:

> [The] nuchal cord is well recognized as being commonly associated with fetal distress and neonatal depression. It is all the more remarkable, therefore, that little work has been published to demonstrate the incidence of the condition, and to analyze its effects during labour and delivery. (Crawford 1962)

This finding was observed in 15% to 30% of nuchal-cord deliveries. Great variances of nuchal-cord observations exist because prenatal diagnosis with ultrasound has only recently been made. The accuracy of previous studies is in question because close adherence to specific definition may not have been followed. Nuchal cords are at the center of the supply-line controversy because so much differing information exists. To study nuchal cords, the fetus involved must be prenatally identified. Cords can wrap around the fetal neck as soon as the cord reaches four-fifths of the fetal length. This occurs as early as ten to twelve weeks' gestational age. Fetuses can entangle themselves multiple times; deliveries of fetuses with six to eight complete loops around the neck have been described. What distinguishes a surviving fetus from a stillborn fetus with a nuchal cord is unclear; however, some insights exist. For example, fetuses born dead with cords around the neck have been described from abortuses (eight to twelve weeks) to postterm (weeks). Yet no one clearly understands when these fetuses die, and no one has clearly observed those cord patterns. Actually, not all nuchal cords are the same. One researcher noticed a predisposition to nuchal-cord-related deaths around thirty-eight weeks. This is difficult to verify because ultrasound was not used to accurately date the fetuses. Another researcher noticed that two patterns exist: the cord crosses over itself, or the cord crosses under itself. This observation may be important when considering knot formations in the cord. A cross-under pattern is needed for knot formation and can cinch a nuchal cord if it rolls back on itself. Are multiple nuchal loops more deadly than single nuchal loops? Does the chance of fetal death increase with the amount of loops in the cord? Again, a definite answer is unknown, but many factors have been noted. Regardless of the number of loops, the problem lies in supply-line disruption. For example, fetuses who are breech are more likely to have more loops than fetuses who are vertex (head down). The shoulders of breech fetuses are freer to rotate than those who are vertex. Placental position is another factor. Activity, again, may influence the formation of nuchal loops. In addition, male infants seem more predisposed than female infants. There are also combinations of these factors. Nuchal cord formation is a function of fetal life. Once a cord is long, it is more likely to affect an active fetus. A very active fetus, especially one with a high level of amniotic fluid volume and a high level of energy derived from placental design, may be predisposed to nuchal cord formation. The number of infants killed by their umbilical cords is unknown. The National Center for Health Statistics does not have enough data to determine this. Possibly as few as four thousand deaths per year or as many as eight thousand deaths per year involve umbilical cord complications. The important point here is, these infants are normal; they are normal, but they are dead. Some researchers believe that cord accidents do not cause death. However, Dr. Arnold Lillien of NICHD explains this may not be correct.

> In general, however, the consensus of opinion has been that a nuchal cord is unlikely to compromise a fetus and is rarely, if ever, a cause of fetal death. We found a significant incidence of

tight nuchal cords among term intrapartum fetal deaths without explanation. (Lillien 1970)

A similar opinion is shared by Torgrim Sørnes, MD, who has studied this issue for two decades. "The pathology of umbilical cord encirclements around the fetal body, neck, or extremities has not been subjected to thorough study for years, and little is known of their etiology, pathogenesis or effects on the fetus." (Sørnes 1995)

Cord Entanglement: The umbilical cord can surround an extremity, the body, or the neck. Body loops can be single or multiple and can exist with nuchal cords. The number of body-loop incidences is unknown. Most of these entanglements are undone at delivery as the infant is being born; therefore, they are never witnessed and never recorded. This lack of documentation in the medical record means, studies that use this information cannot be accurate. To date, PI's PUCP has this data.

The effect of a body loop is cord compression. Tight loops have made impressions on the skin of the fetus and can restrict fetal movement in the uterus. Loops around the extremity can affect circulation of the extremity and cause damage to a foot or a hand. Circulation disturbances can sometimes form blood clots in the arteries, vein, or placenta. These events can change the oxygen supply to the fetus and cause growth disturbances or death. Yet the variety and magnitude of cord entanglement become evident when one considers factors such as cord design, Wharton's jelly thickness, placental types, cord insertion sites, and fetal position. The explanation is not impossible and may be finite. There are no prenatally derived statistics that can provide the scope and incidence of cord entanglement. To arrive at this explanation, an understanding is needed of the number of prenatal incidences, the length of time that nonnuchal-cord entanglement lasts, and the effects on the fetus.

Combinations:

These experiments show that even a slack knot may be sufficient to interfere with, if not completely obstruct, the cord circulation, but that any pull upon the knot such as might be exerted if the cord were wound around the child's neck or body as to cause a relative shortening of it, would easily cause sufficient tightening to impede the circulation completely.

—Francis J. Browne, MD
Edinburgh Royal Maternity Hospital
Great Britain, 1923

Three cases of umbilical cord entanglement were described as complex (combinations). The cases were associated with intermittent fetal bradycardia, reduced fetal movements, and prematurely delivery. Umbilical cord loops were around the neck, limbs, and body. Placental pathology showed downstream effects of cord occlusion and fetal thrombotic vasculopathy.

M Dodds, R Windim, J Kingdom
Ontario, Canada 2012

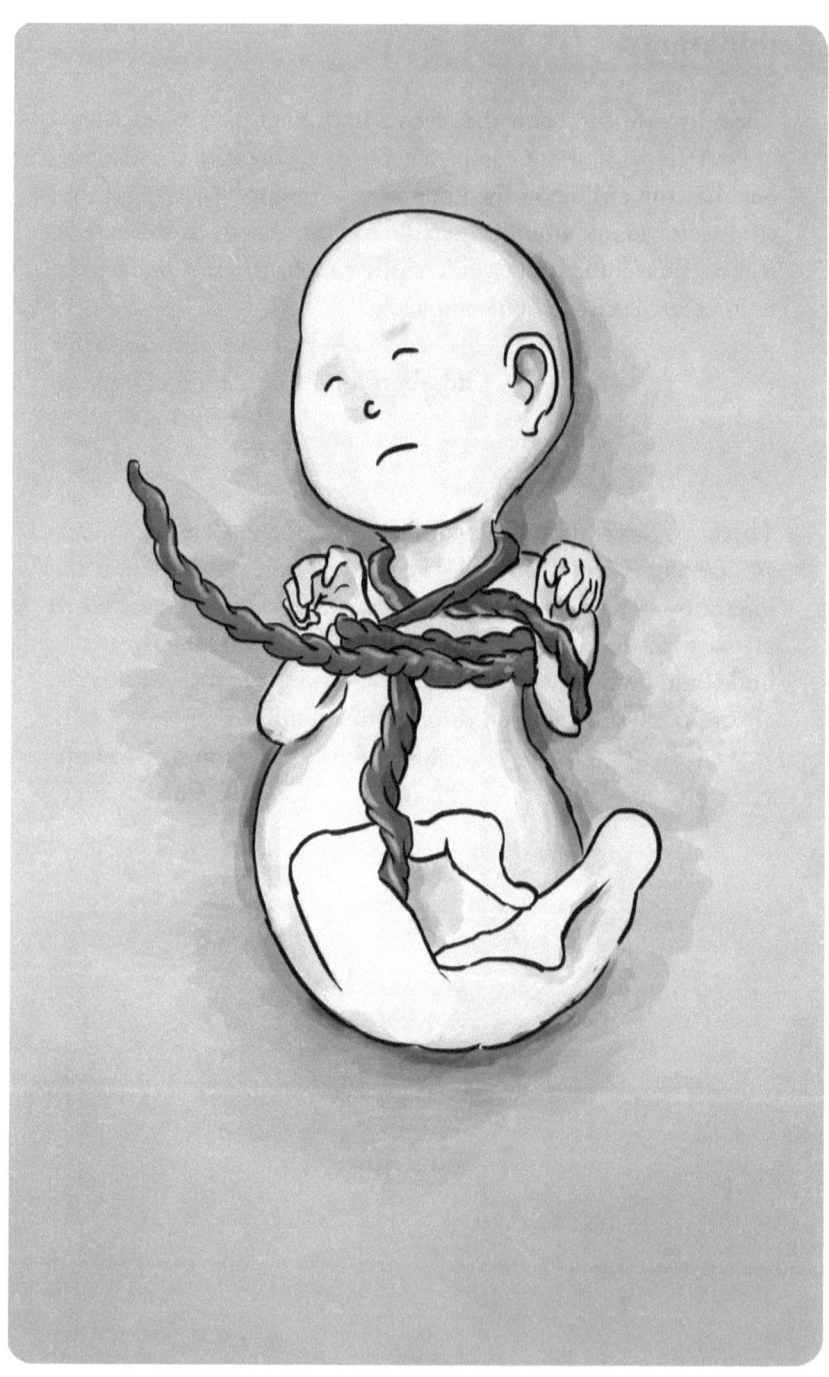

Combination UCA

In addition to individual cord conditions creating fetal disturbances, potentially dangerous combinations are often observed. Yet the risk of harm is unknown. Whether a combined cord complication increases the chance of stillbirth compared to a single cord complication is unknown.

Another unknown is the effect the mother's toxemia or a disorder such as anemia may have on the fetus. Combinations involving fetal umbilical cord insertion-site hematomas (vessel rupture) have been observed. These hematomas were associated with nuchal loops, true knots, and midcord hematomas. These particular combinations suggest an umbilical cord subject to stretch mechanisms, possibly tearing the umbilical vein near its insertion. Reports of infants born with more than one knot and as many as three imply that fetal activity and repositioning are key factors. Were all three knots formed at once or one at a time? Is there a time during fetal development that is at highest risk for multiple knot formation?

The gestational age at which knots form would be valuable information so that increased screening could be initiated at that gestational age. Infants delivered with nuchal cords and a true knot are not uncommon. Upon closer inspection, the cord is usually long. The excessive length increases the probability of knot formation, but it is not necessarily deadly. Increased slack decreases the chance of tension. Cord architecture is also a factor. However, in studies that recorded length, cord type was not included.

Torsion: Torsion is the condition of the umbilical cord where twists are superimposed on the cord itself. Knots and nuchal cords are not always seen with torsion, but they can be observed with torsion. This combination, though, can be dangerous because cord positions that allow tension will cause torsioned cords to kink. Torsion is tolerable as long as the torque (imposed twist force) is released as a deformation of the cord (a snarl). If the energy of the snarl is reimposed, the cord blocks just like a garden hose. A deadly combination is a cord under torsion with a shoulder loop, nuchal cord, body loop, or extremity loop.

Finding vessel thrombus combined with torsion is not unusual. These thrombi can also be seen in the surface vessels of the placenta. Many of these combinations go unnoticed simply because no one is looking for them. When blockage occurs with cord-compression mechanisms, one of the clues left behind is edema (a buildup of fluid) of the cord. It is not unusual, for example, to have a nuchal cord with proximal cord edema, suggesting mild episodes of blood flow disturbance but not enough to cause death. In addition, it is not unusual for these combinations to cause fetal heart rate changes severe enough during labor to cause an emergency C-section. Short cords may be more dangerous because they are shorter, may marginally attach, and may be a velamentous insertion. This increases the chances of umbilical cord rupture compared to a normal insertion. Short cords may also predispose the cord vessels to thrombosis, hemorrhage, or hematoma formation. Individual reports of such occurrences are published in the medical literature. Although not common individually, all combinations as a whole present a significant occurrence when viewed on a larger scale. When combined, these events represent a more prevalent failure of reproductive mechanisms when compared to the most common genetic malformations. Altogether, in any community hospital practicing obstetrics, cord complications will be observed more often than congenital defects.

For instance, one medical review of just hematoma formation of the umbilical cord at Johns Hopkins Medical Center was observed in 1 out of 5,505 cases. Down Syndrome, a common genetic alteration known as trisomy 21 syndrome, occurs overall as 1 in every 660 deliveries. Trisomy 18, another readily acquired genetic defect, occurs as 1 in every 3,000 deliveries. Trisomy 13 occurs as 1 in every 5,000 deliveries.

Hematoma of the Umbilical Cord:

> The causes of rupture of an umbilical vessel are obscure and probably several factors enter into the development of a hematoma in each case.
> —A. Louis Dippel, MD
> Johns Hopkins University and Hospital
> Baltimore, Maryland, 1940

A hematoma of the umbilical cord is due to bleeding into the substance of the umbilical cord. They can be spontaneous, iatrogenically induced, traumatic self-induced, or secondary to an umbilical cord defect. The usual risk of cord hematomas that is often quoted is 1/1,000 to 1/5,500 rps deliveries. Hematomas can be due to the umbilical artery or umbilical vein. This sausage-shaped injury seems to be more frequently noticed on the fetal end than on the placental end. The chance of death to the fetus is as high as 50% and as low as 14%. The cause of hematoma development is unknown. Some scientific insights suggest wearing of the vessel walls, thinning of the walls, tearing, and then bleeding into the substance of the cord. Compression of the cord vessels leads to clogging and then death of the fetus. The sight of hematoma formation can vary, however. Again, unknowns exist in the area of umbilical cord hematomas. For example, it is unclear whether the cause of the fetal-end hematoma is the same as the placental-end hematoma. The most common time of hematoma formation is also unknown. Most discussions of formation have centered around labor and delivery. This would suggest that cord tension may play a role, and this tension can possibly be attributed to a condition where the cord is stretched. Obviously, observation of this condition was recognized long before recorded history and must have motivated many speculations. Since most modern reports (1871 to present) have described mostly stillborns, cord compression is an end result. Numerous descriptions focus on hematomas that originate from the umbilical skin. Vessels penetrating the Wharton's jelly from the umbilicus may rupture from fetal manipulation, which includes pulling on the umbilical insertion. Infants can grasp before birth and have been observed sucking and pulling on everything in the uterine amniotic cavity.

The most difficult feature of umbilical cord hematomas is that they are spontaneous and evolve quickly. Many case descriptions suggest that the fetuses were not in labor. More information is needed about the timing of these events and particular fetal behavior that may predispose the cord to hematomas if the fetus is vulnerable.

Torsion: As previously described, torsion is the condition of the umbilical cord where twists are superimposed on the cord itself, similar to an overly twisted telephone cord.

Umbilical cord torsion may not be an unusual finding. "In human beings, the umbilical cord is subject to many kinds of torsion, coiling, looping and knotting during pregnancy or during parturition. Torsion of the cord is a common occurrence." (Atwood 1932)

No formal definition of torsion currently exists. Veterinary scientific literature is quite familiar with the problem of torsion, especially in thoroughbreds. In fact, torsion is often a cause of fetal loss in horses. Veterinarians readily observe this finding and look for confirmation by studying other fetal structures confirming its presence as the cause of death. In one study of fetal losses in horses, 200/2,000 were due to this umbilical cord accident. Another topic more easily discussed in animal research is the association of torsion with heart failure and the finding of thromboses in the placenta. Clearly, torsion is readily accepted as a cause of fetal death in animals. For humans, this is not the perception. Some think that torsion occurs after death as a result of random movements of the dead fetus.

Prior to the Pregnancy Institute's study of torsion of the umbilical cord, no case report of a live birth with torsion existed in the medical literature. All descriptions of human umbilical cord-related torsion have been in stillborns. Therefore, the Pregnancy Institute's information did not come about easily. Dr. Kurt Benirschke, a Harvard-trained pathologist and professor emeritus of pathology at the University of California, San Diego, has provided us with invaluable insights into the mystery of this fetal/placental abnormality, especially torsion of the umbilical cord. He determined that the cord becomes intensely twisted, placental damage occurs secondary to thromboses, a common time of death is between twenty-eight and thirty weeks' gestational age, and torsion of the umbilical cord is seen in cerebral palsy cases. With this information, our observations of umbilical cord torsion began with normal live deliveries. Dr. Benirschke's suggestion of an intensely twisted umbilical cord prompted us to untwist the cord in over four hundred deliveries. We determined that torsion is actually very common but not always pathologic. Next, we determined the time in which pathology occurs and the spectrum of effects. The effect of torsion can be fetal harm ranging from heart failure to stillbirth. Torsion is not a natural state of the umbilical cord. Torsioned cords must not be confused with naturally helical, coiled, or spiraled cords. The appropriate terminology should be the word *helical*, which implies a constant, if not same, diameter. Torsion and natural helixes are different from each other. According to European literature, the curly course of the cord was considered in 1521, and left versus right (clockwise/counterclockwise) patterns were recognized in the 1600s. Left curls (80%) predominate over right curls (20%). Early estimates of total curls averaged eleven turns per cord (Hyrtl 1890). These estimates may be different from each other, however, because twists were not removed by unwinding. Most umbilical cords on the average (55 cm) have three to five helixes, the upper limit having eight helixes. The average number of twists is three. Together, the average curls could be Hyrtl's eleven. These same quantities are also found in equine cords. Cords can become twisted when the fetus repositions itself. Therefore, torsion is not an umbilical cord anomaly or abnormality. It is a mechanical deformation/alteration due to the behavior of the fetus. The importance of the formation of torsion implies much about intrauterine life and the dangers that face the fetus. These dangers are as significant as those that a newborn gazelle faces on the African savannah. The fetus begins to move around ten weeks' gestational age. If fetal activity is excessive, trouble begins. Torsion, nuchal-cord formation, body-loop formation, and true knots are related. The relationship depends on the type of repositioning that takes place. Fetuses can tumble, roll, and somersault like a gymnast in the three-dimensional environment. Torsion occurs when the fetus imparts these motions to the cord. This mechanical energy is called torque and is subject to the same laws of physics as any structure that is deformed by the same force. Twists occur as a result of this torque, and torsion occurs when twists involve every ninth a ratio of 1 twist per 5 cm or less of cord length. Torsion of the cord is a remarkable example of nature on the edge. For example, if a 50-cm cord has 10 twists imparted to it by thirty weeks, it can relieve the torque by growth of the cord. If the fetus remains in one position after thirty weeks, the cord could grow another 10 cm and change from a ratio of 1 twist to 5 cm (1/5) to 1 twist to 6 cm (1/6). The danger is therefore averted.

Collapse and kinking of the cord blood vessels seem to occur at a ratio below 1/5. The cord must then stretch so it can redistribute the stress/strain of the torque, which usually ends up being at a point near the placental end of the cord. A simple example is a telephone cord. Once heavily twisted, it narrows and snarls (loops over itself). Over time it becomes a complete mess. Torsion is an umbilical cord complication that is dependent on a number of factors. For example, fetal behavior is determined by intrauterine needs. This intrauterine fetal ballet has a purpose, function, and plan: get the fetus into a comfortable head-down prelabor position. The fetus may attempt this several times before reaching the milestone. Its success within a few attempts depends on placental position, amniotic fluid volume, inner ear (vestibular) maturation, and maternal diet and activity. If one of these factors is exaggerated, the fetus may begin the process of excessive activity, continued repositioning, and torque of the umbilical cord.

> Undue twisting of the cord (torsion not coiling), especially in that portion near the fetus where the Wharton's jelly is less abundant, probably can cause feta asphyxia. In the case illustrated, death of the fetus occurred about a week before delivery and was preceded by a period of *violent movements*. (Novak 1941)

Because torsion and its effects are also dependent on umbilical cord length, short cords may succumb faster than longer cords. Again, the type of cord may also play a role where type IV (vein around arteries) may be more prone to collapse under equal stress than other types (arteries around vein). Cord diameter/circumference also plays a role. A thicker cord may offer more resistance to torque than a thin cord. This is in need of study and will require a specialized vascular laboratory. Fetuses may also possess natural reflexes that allow them to untwist themselves. Cord helixes can be left and right in nature but mostly left (80%). If the fetus counterpositions itself, under favorable conditions of intrauterine life, it can get itself out of a perilous torsion. How often and in what way the fetus repositions itself during intrauterine life are unknown. One clue to this question is the twists seen at delivery. We have found that the average number of twists is $3\frac{1}{2}$. This was determined by untwisting over 300 umbilical cords at birth. It suggests that the fetus repositions itself in one direction 360 degrees ($3^1/_2$ revolutions). Unfortunately, the fetus may move in clockwise and counterclockwise directions. This would suggest that 6 moves left to right could be negated by 3 moves right to left, leaving the 3 twists as an inaccurate record. The fetus probably moves more often in the same direction and usually does not reposition itself often. Ideally, a constant series of ultrasound exams or a device that detects fetal position (like global positioning systems) might give us the final answer. Knowledge of the usual intrauterine activity over time would help solve the problem of torsion. [Insight—skin reference which would be trackable.]

Umbilical Cord Knots:

> The number of knots on the umbilical cord of a first born child is held to foretell how many of a family the mother is to have.
> —"Umbilical Cord Folklore"
> *The British Medical Journal*
> 1912

On first inspection, it is remarkable that a fetus can tie a knot in its umbilical cord. How is that possible? Monoamniotic twins (twins in the same sac) can create multiple knots together. No reports, however, exist that Siamese twins had knots in their common cord. This twin anomaly of reproduction suggests that the fetus must move to form a knot. Two separate fetuses moving independently create cord chaos, which can lead to multiple sites of constriction and fetal death. So how does a knot form, and what happens to the knot in utero? Most true knots are probably not formed before birth but during birth. It is highly likely that the fetus is entangled with the cord and, when delivered, is pulled through a loop of cord, forming a knot. To form a knot, the loop of cord must be special. It must be long enough for the fetus to form a nuchal cord. The nuchal cord must cross under itself, not over itself. This cross-under pattern allows the formation of a single hitch knot. The loop of crossed-under nuchal cord must pass over the fetal body before a knot can form. This specialized loop sometimes forms around an ankle and entraps it. The fetus is born with a snared ankle instead of a true knot. Sometimes both ankles can be involved. If the knot completes itself, the risk of blockage is great. We speculate that prenatal knots may form prior to thirty-two weeks, a common time of fetal repositioning. Yet the time at which most knots form prenatally is unknown. Knots may form earlier and have been noted prior to twenty weeks in miscarriage specimens. The earliest knot seen prenatally with ultrasound is in monoamniotic twins at nineteen weeks.

To envision knot formation, it is important to remember torsion. As the fetus repositions in the uterus, it applies torque to the umbilical cord; this energy causes the cord to loop counter to the direction of the torque, thereby crossing counter to the fetal movements. A cross-under loop has now formed, which, if lassoed around the fetal neck, can work its way along the fetal body to form a knot. The fetus may not even have to change position because its movements may work the loop to its feet and then off. Knot complexity depends on the amount of snarls created at the base of the loop. One snarl creates a single knot, two snarls a double knot, and three or more snarls a complex knot. Double snarls with double loops have also been described. The whole process is actually simple. A complex knot does not imply multiple fetal tumbles and twists. It only means the fetus passed through a loop or loops simultaneously. How the fetus can cinch a knot tight and block blood supply depends on other factors. As with a prolapsed cord, complete compression of blood flow will cause fetal harm. A knot can completely block the cord, and a knot can be tightened by the fetus during prenatal life. The chance of having a fetus deliver with a true knot of the umbilical cord is on the average 1% to 2%. The chance of fetal demise secondary to a knot blockage is 5% to 10%. It is not known whether the most common knot is a single, double, or triple knot. It is also unknown whether more complex knots are more deadly. It is known, however, that the chance of fetal death is increased with a knotted cord.

Body/Extremity Loops: Body and extremity loops, some of the more difficult mechanisms to observe, may be significant causes of fetal decompensation. Anecdotal reports have described extremities damaged by tight loops. The ability of these loops to injure an arm or leg but not cause fetal death is difficult to determine. Stillbirths are observed with multiple loops around ankles, necks, and bodies; yet it is difficult to determine which compressed segment caused death. Cord loops around the body are usually not observed because delivery unwraps them. The loop puzzle is pulled apart at the moment of delivery, so it goes unseen. The incidence seen at delivery is probably less than what actually takes place prenatally over time; probably 0.5% to 2% is reported. The increased chance of stillbirth is still debated. Chinese and Russian medical literatures tend to suggest that loops are not benign. If a fetus persists with a body loop, the chance of cord compression appears greater than if no loop exists. Body loops also can act like winches, taking up slack and causing relative shortness of the cord. This shortness may lead to placental separation and, in one report, maternal amniotic fluid embolism. Does a fetus recognize that its supply line is being compressed? Is there a fetal instinct that reacts to limitation of movement? Currently, some basic science experiments in rats suggest that this exists. Observations of entangled fetuses suggest the fetus is moving in one direction and not back and forth. Untangling a triple nuchal cord is usually in the same clockwise or counterclockwise direction in which it formed. Most loops originate over the fetal right shoulder and unwind counterclockwise. Similarly, torsion untwists clockwise. Fetuses may instinctively be preprogrammed to register favorable right-to-left rolls.

Whether this is totally reflex, chance, or instinctive evasive movements is unknown. The role of the inner ear (balance, orientation) vestibular system is also unknown. Could the fetus become faint or dizzy in utero? If so, does this cause unusual fetal movements that lead to tumbles/somersaults and rolls? Can diet play a role? It is suggested that caffeine and xanthines (tobacco, chocolate, tea, coffee, soft drinks) may keep the fetus awake. Does this predispose the fetus to more activity and possibly more risk? Does the fetus develop a sense of position as well? After all, fetal hearing matures around twenty-four weeks. The fetus hears low-frequency sounds. The vestibular system is an ancient, evolutionary sense. Fish have had it for a long time. Is the fetus using its well-developed sense of position since its taste, smell, and sight senses cannot determine its orientation? If so, can its sense of position be disrupted by other stimuli and send it into a search pattern of disoriented movement resulting in body loops? How cord compression affects the fetus is discussed in the next chapter. How the fetus behaves and why it may be designed not to entangle itself will also be addressed next.

It is suggested that the reduced fetal movements and the changes in fetal heart rate were due to a diminished blood flow in the cord vessels as a result of gradual cord compression. (Sadovski 1976)

Three umbilical cord complications occur at least once in every four deliveries, and their problem cannot be avoided. (Spellacy 1966)

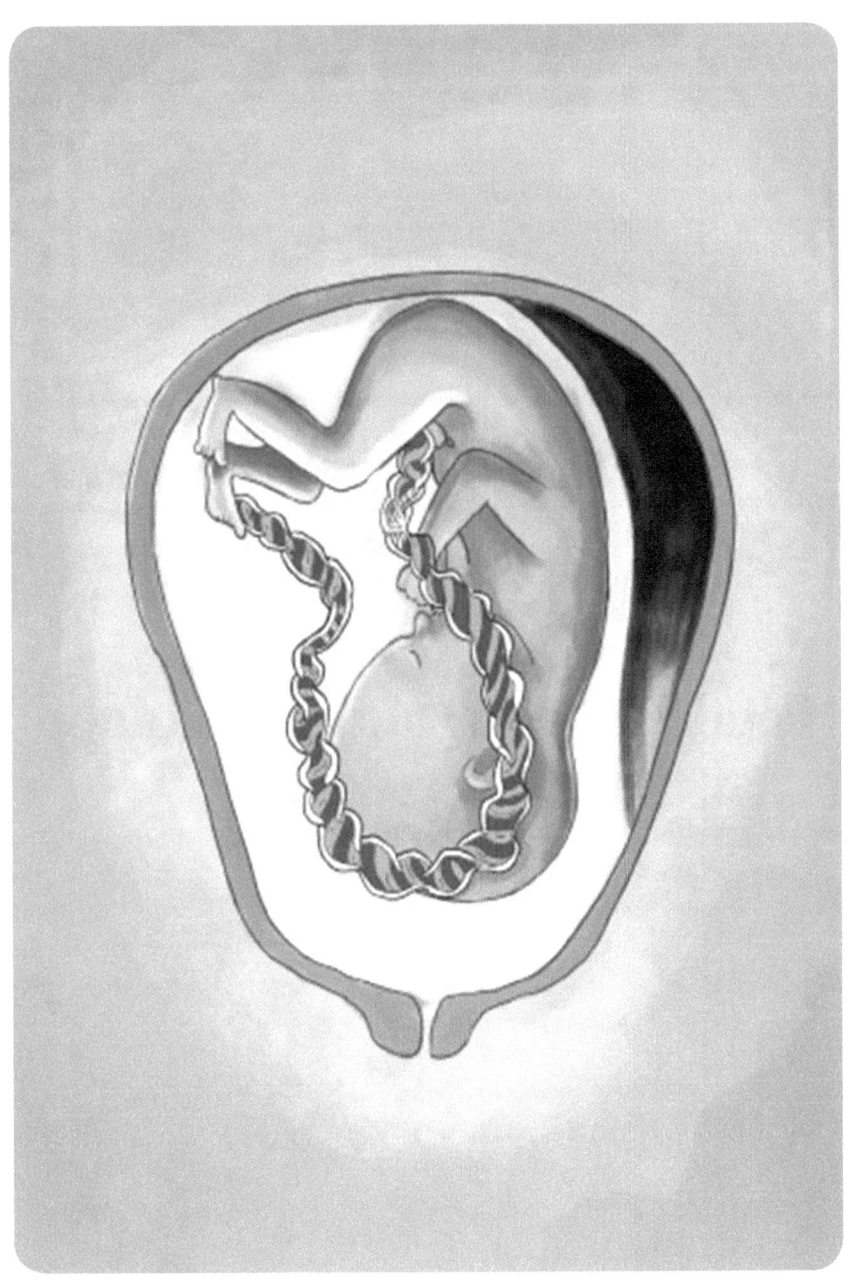
Umbilical Cord Compression

CHAPTER THREE

Fetal Behavior and Physiology

Whatever may be the final determination concerning the etiology of coiling of the cord, the movements of the foetus will undoubtedly play a prominent part in it.
—John Paterson Gardiner, MD
Toledo, Ohio,
1922

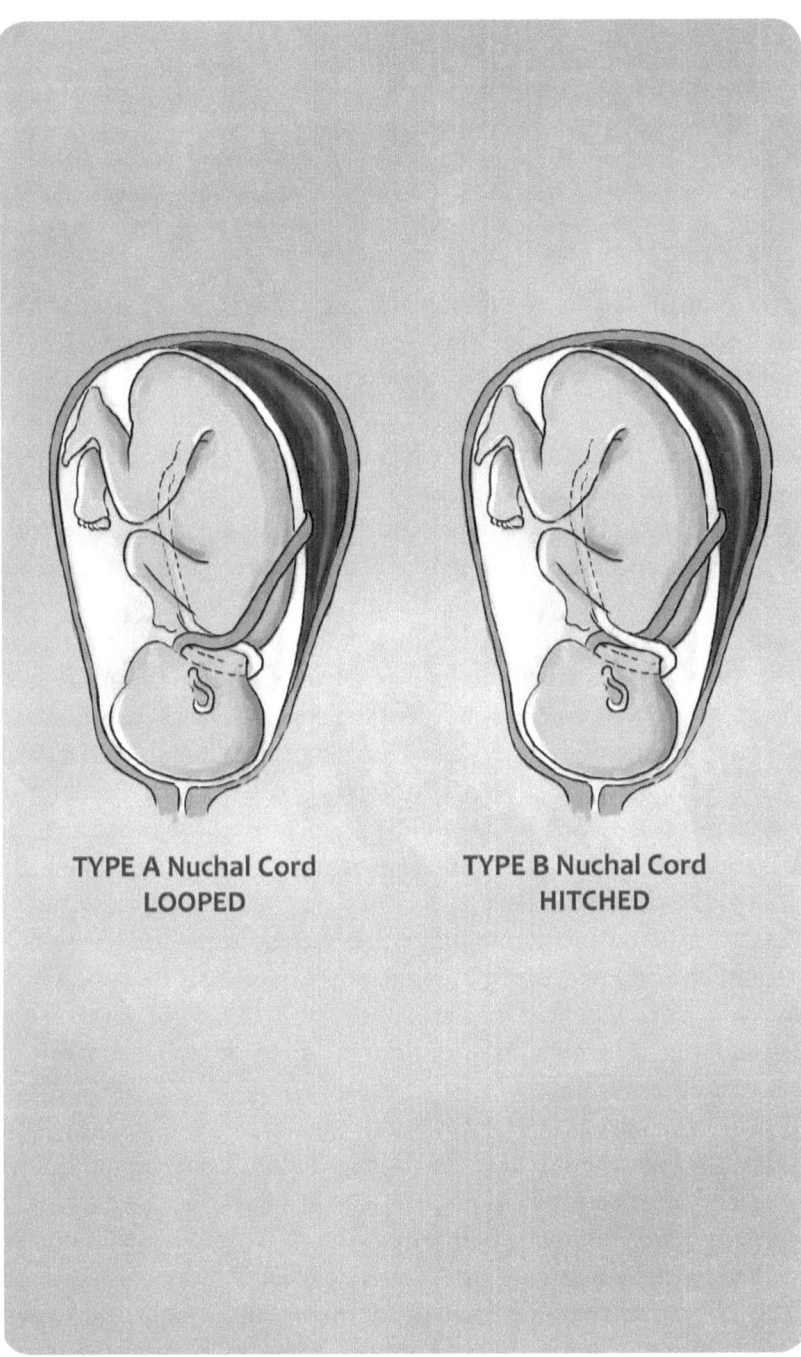

**TYPE A Nuchal Cord
LOOPED**

**TYPE B Nuchal Cord
HITCHED**

> Any fetus that frequently changes position as found by routine examination is a candidate for torsion, looping, or knotting of the cord.
>
> —James P. Hennessy, MD
> New York, New York,
> 1964

Before the invention of ultrasound technology, much uncertainty surrounded the unseen developing fetus. How the fetus grows, moves, sleeps, and acts in the uterus was not certain. Ultrasonography allowed visualization of the fetus inside the mother as it transforms itself up to the moment of labor and delivery. Visually studying these behaviors has allowed for new insights. Fetal heart rate monitoring is the detection and recording of the fetus's beat-to-beat heart rate. This noninvasive electronic tool allows study of fetal reaction to its intrauterine environment under stressful conditions. Changes in the quality and character of the beat-to-beat pattern of the fetal heart allow graphic patterns to be recorded that translate into some basic fetal physiologic conditions. Fetal heart rate monitoring and ultrasound imaging together have contributed to the overall impression obstetricians have today of how the fetus works and interacts with the placenta, umbilical cord, uterus, and mother. Dr. Peter Nathanielsz, MD, PhD, has studied fetal development for the National Institutes of Health. He states, "Ultrasound shows us that each fetus has his or her own personality . . . . We can use ultrasound as a video camera on the developing fetus. We can track the fetus's heart beat and can follow his responses to sound and uterine contractures (uterine cramps which last 5 minutes) . . . . Ultrasound reveals the intricate systems which have evolved to allow human survival and continuation of life."

3-D and 4-D ultrasounds have the ability to view the fetus in more detail. More than thirty umbilical cord pathologies have been documented in peer-reviewed imaging literature. A new imaging tool, the MRI (magnetic resonance imaging), can also identify these pathologies. Ideally, the current eighteen—to twenty-week ultrasound study should include the fetus, placenta, and umbilical cord. It should state the placental position, site of cord attachment, type and length of umbilical cord (twisted versus straight), and fetal umbilical cord attachment.

RECOMMENDED READING

Comprehensive imaging review of abnormalities of the umbilical cord. *Moshiri M[1], Zaidi SF, Robinson TJ, Bhargava P, Siebert JR, Dubinsky TJ, Katz DS. Radiographics.* 2014 Jan-Feb;34(1):179-96.

To understand the fetal ballet of intrauterine life, a place to start is the shape of the uterus itself. The uterus is neither globular nor cylindrical but bean-shaped. The bulge is created by the lower back (spine) as it bends forward (lordosis at 2 cm-4 cm) with pregnancy. Lordosis creates a central hump in the uterus that helps stabilize the fetus from excessive motion. It may serve as an obstacle to fetal rolling. Finally, this shape may guide the fetus to a head-down launch position by thirty-seven weeks.

Throughout pregnancy, this choreographed, instinctive behavior is directly linked to fetal survival. The fetus develops intrauterine reflexes to cope with maternal movements and positions. Without these abilities, the fetus will fail in its journey to birth. A new perspective on the fetus that is at odds with the old perspective has emerged in the last thirty years. The fetus is believed to be independent of the mother relative to its behavior. The fetus is also believed to control the onset of labor through its own local biochemistry, such as its endocrine and paracrine systems. These scientific facts put forth a view that the fetus is like a tadpole in a pond. Amphibian eggs are laid and left to fend for themselves. The tadpole develops independent of the mother through multiple stages. The human fetus develops in the pond called the uterus without any direct maternal care. It must fend for itself. Thus, the fetus is an active participant in its development and environment, and it decides when it is born. It signals the mom to initiate labor, and part of that process is causing the release of melatonin from the maternal pineal gland from 9:00 p.m. to 6:00 a.m. This release is directly connected to uterine contractions, which is why most natural deliveries are at night. The fetus reaches milestones in the uterus just as a newborn reaches milestones of rolling, crawling, and walking over time. This scientific philosophy of fetal life points to behavior mechanisms of the fetus that would allow instinctive protection of the supply line (umbilical cord) by inherent reflexes. Evolutionary changes had to favor a combination of relative relationships that would allow success of a reproductive assembly such as ours. Mammalian species all have cord-related complications. Monkeys, horses, alpacas, and cattle have all been observed with umbilical cord problems. One difference is that these animals must be prepared to fend for themselves and ambulate at birth. The human is dependent at birth but is somewhat independent in the uterus. Cord compression can occur in the uterus. If labor begins (Braxton-Hicks contractions that can take three weeks), cord compression can intensify. The fetus can adapt to mild, infrequent cord compression and can resolve it. This can be observed using ultrasound, especially in pregnancies with multiple siblings, large uterine fibroids, and abnormal placental cord insertions, such as velamentous insertions and low-lying posterior insertions. This umbilical cord compression has associated reflexes and has been observed in animal models during controlled laboratory experiments. These experiments in pregnant rats and sheep fetuses that reproduce cord compression have observed fetal jerking movements, hiccups, and change of fetal position, which are believed to relieve the site of umbilical cord compression. These movements have been observed in human fetuses. It is believed that human single fetuses respond to cord compression with these reflexes. A type of human fetal-jerking movement has been described as a hiccup. These movements are rhythmical and last for ten to fifteen minutes. There should be two to three episodes in a twenty-four-hour period.

Dr. Joseph B. DeLee, professor of obstetrics, Northwestern University Medical School, wrote in his 1913 *Principles and Practice of Obstetrics* that hiccups were one of the most interesting phenomena of intrauterine life. The movements are short, quick jerks of the shoulders and trunk. In connection with these observations, he wrote that it was impossible to be sure that the infant was not suffering from asphyxia and was gasping for breath.

A later observer of this behavior was researcher John Patrick, MD (Toronto, Canada), who studied hiccups with ultrasound. He believed that three to four fifteen-minute hiccup episodes in twenty-four hours were normal. These episodes are observed beginning at twenty-six weeks and are diminished after thirty-two weeks. Hiccups are minimized toward term. A fetus having hiccups at term should be investigated. Do not assume frequent hiccups are OK.

A recent observation by Osamu Kurauchi, MD, of Nagoya, Japan, School of Medicine, supports the idea that startling, jumping, and writhing movements should diminish as the fetus matures. Studying anencephalic fetuses (without brains), he observed that as the fully formed brain matures, these activities are modified, and the behavior lessened toward term. In 1750, Dr. Smellie observed an infant with cord entanglement experiencing hiccups during vaginal delivery and afterward. We have reported that hiccups after three to four episodes lasting less than fifteen minutes in a twenty-four-hour period may not be physiologic and that more than three to four hiccup episodes occurring during maternal activity may suggest cord compression.

The nerve impulses that may cause hiccups may originate by way of the umbilical ring (belly button). Cholinergic and adrenergic nerve terminals, or end nests, have been identified in the umbilical cord 20 cm out and concentrated toward the umbilical ring. These nerve fibers run with the umbilical vein and sacral plexus to join the phrenic ganglion and celiac ganglion in proximity to the ductus venosus. The ductus venosus controls blood flow into the liver from the umbilical vein. It contains nerves and monitors fetal physiology. These fibers run with the vagal trunks and eventually may interact with the phrenic nerve by way of the medulla and respiratory center. The phrenic nerve sends fibers to the pericardium, phrenic ganglion, sympathetic plexus, and hepatic plexus. Compression or stretch of the umbilical cord may lead to spasm of the ductus venosus and contractions of the diaphragm similar to a reflex. This activity may be originating at the umbilical ring, which may be a pressure/blood flow sensor. These nerve pathways are basic structures of the human body and how it senses basic body functions. Fetal behavior is directly linked to its physiology and is based on reflexes (like an eye blink for dust irritation).

The way the fetus conserves oxygen, glucose, and water and its reaction to these altered elements are remarkable adaptations of an interactive life as compared to a more dependent development. The fetus is constantly faced with a changing physical compartment called the uterus. As the fetus grows and expands, it first encounters a cavity that is twice its size. Between implantation and twelve weeks, the fetus (embryo) remains on a short cord tether, thick and restrictive to motion; it also repositions and reacts to maternal activity. The fetus, therefore, is stable relative to its position. This is not the case after twelve weeks. As the uterus grows and the cavity becomes several times larger than the fetus by amniotic fluid expansion, the fetus now has "wings," extended arms and legs that are movable. Maternal activity can now distort fetal stability, and the fetus must respond to it or risk its supply line. Imagine an astronaut in space working on the space shuttle and spinning out of control. The line connecting life support to the shuttle will eventually fail. In intrauterine space, the fetus must develop a means to orient itself to react to maternal movements. This is accomplished by growth; fetal extremities resisting spin, roll, and tumble; and fetal reflexes adjusting fetal position. As the fetus matches uterine growth between twenty weeks and thirty-two weeks, fetal reflex responses and mass act like a disc brake to grab the intrauterine anatomy to stay put. The fetus can exercise and develop, but it is able to remain stationary and not reposition itself (similar to working a treadmill). There is a difference between fetal movements and fetal motion (repositioning). The fetus is designed not to roll, spin, or tumble because these motions are deadly. Fetal physiology as it applies to behavior of the fetus is primarily working to prepare the fetus for birth. It must have the ability to respond to changes that affect its heart rate, metabolic rate, neurologic status, and position. These alterations are the sources of fetal surveillance on which obstetricians depend to determine whether the fetus is compromised.

Fetal Senses

The main fetal senses are vision, hearing, touch, taste, and smell. Vision while developing is limited in utero. Eyelids are closed up until twenty-six weeks. Whether the fetus perceives light is unclear. At birth, newborns perceive shadows but do not clearly distinguish shapes. Vision would appear to be neither a primary mechanism for fetal behavior nor a means for the fetus to determine its position and status. In adults, vision is very important for day/night signals that manufacture melatonin and influence circadian rhythms. Fetal rhythms may be determined by maternal behavior and when meals are eaten.

Smell is not well developed at birth nor is taste, which depends on smell. Nose plugs exist during fetal life; therefore, smell would not determine how a fetus presents itself. Chemical markers are important to many animal species for identifying food, dangers, and each other. Yet for human fetuses, smell does not appear to play a major role in the uterus. Fetuses do not appear to identify parents by sight or smell at first. There is no need to forage for food in the uterus. Smell and taste only appear necessary in extrauterine life. Swallowing, however, is connected to intrauterine and extrauterine life. The fetus must swallow fluid to make urine and develop the gastrointestinal tract. Suggestions indicate that what the mother ingests may reach these fetal senses through the bloodstream. This backdoor chemosensory smell effect could play a role in how or whether the fetus ingests amniotic fluid.

What does amniotic fluid taste like to the fetus? Is the taste covered up by the chemosensory effects, like putting sauce on a steak? These answers are unknown; yet whatever the purpose, it is probable that these senses do not have the same role in intrauterine life. They may play a role in initiating labor by responding to meconium discharged to the amniotic fluid. Meconium is the product of the fetal intestines, which turns amniotic fluid green when expelled. Because meconium contains bile acids and other chemicals, ingestion may stimulate nerve receptors in the fetal nose and throat. These fetal nerve endings may contribute to neurologic signals reaching the hypothalamus, initiating the onset of labor. Touch is an important sense for the fetus. Our knowledge of fetal touch is understood by what we know about newborns. The rooting reflex appears to develop after birth. Before birth, this sense appears to work in the opposite way. For example, a fetus seen on ultrasound turns away when touched on the cheek. Sucking fingers, toes, and umbilical cords have also been observed on ultrasound. Yet turning away may be protective. Cord sucking may cause cord compression. In the uterus, turning away from objects may be beneficial. Touching and feeling the uterus, placenta, umbilical cord, and bony pelvis must be a part of fetal development. It may be a means for the fetus to locate comfort zones. Yet this may be more a function of pressure sensation than of feel sensation. It is believed that the fetus can feel at different degrees from head to toe. The head is more "sense mature" than the lower body and extremities. The fetus probably prefers to feel itself and spends a lot of time touching with its hands. Fetal grasping is reflex oriented. It is unknown how strong fetal grasp is (how much pressure it exerts). Can the fetus squeeze hard enough with its hand to occlude its umbilical cord with a pressure of 60 mm Hg or greater? It is also unknown whether touch or pressure influences fetal position. Hearing and position (vestibular) senses are related.

Another parallel sense is called kinesthetic sense or "Where are my body parts?" These neurologic developments are the results of millions of years of evolution. The oldest sense is vestibular (inner ear). Even before the appearance of man, fish have had a position sense. It is not known whether the fetus senses gravity, weight, and orientation. The nerves to the ear mature around twenty-four to twenty-six weeks. At this point, the fetus can hear low-frequency noises. It recognizes the maternal voice at birth. It may also have a sense of gravity (up/down). What role does hearing play in the uterus? Although the answer is unknown, we do know that the fetus can be startled with sounds in the uterus. These startle reflexes may play a role in controlling fetal position. Known startle reflexes, such as the Moro reflex, are usually described after birth. This pattern of fetal movement is well known and can be seen by shaking a newborn. The arms take on a hug position with the hands going out away from the body then inward.

What does this reflex look like inside the uterus? Imagine it as a fetal brake. The mother moves suddenly, and the fetus reaches outward to create contact between the uterus and itself. This has been observed on ultrasound, with the mother standing and lying. There are other startle-reflex patterns and fetal movements called tonic neck reflex, which extend the fetal arm, the opposite leg, and the head turns toward the extended arm. These reflexes are not intentional fetal movements as the fetus does not have coordinated movements. However, these movements do have an effect on helping the fetus change position. The vestibular mechanism may be connected to the startle reflexes to position the fetus and provide a means of avoiding cord entanglement. Neural systems connected to the kidneys and related to the midsection play a role in posturing independent of the spinal-cord input. These extravestibular gravity receptors may also be connected to the cardiovascular system through a major nerve called the vagus nerve. This connection is very important to fetal stability. Auditory senses may assist in neurologic development for birth and help provide parent recognition. How would these senses work to protect the fetus when it is active and asleep? When the fetus moves, it does so by movement of the midsection and the neck. These muscle groups are stronger than the extremities. It is often observed that the fetus kicks and jumps in utero. These activities are not coordinated and are not deliberately initiated by the fetus. When the fetus repositions itself as opposed to movements, different factors are involved. For example, the fetus may sense inner-ear pressure, which may change with position; the fetus may sense contours and prefer the left lateral position. In addition, auditory awareness of the placental souffle or maternal heartbeat may predispose the fetus to the head-down/left-lateral position. When uncomfortable, the fetus may attempt to roll, tumble, or somersault, using its startle reflexes to find comfort. This becomes more difficult after thirty-two weeks as the fetus is now larger than the uterine cavity and must fold itself into a fetal posture. If, in the process of repositioning, the baby becomes cord entangled, it may sense this through resistance to movement or the consequences of disturbed blood flow, oxygenation, and nutrient delivery.

Fetal Physiology as It Relates to Cord Compression

When the umbilical cord is compressed, the fetus immediately senses it. If the compression persists, the fetus will begin to undergo heart rate changes. These changes are sensed chemically (chemoreceptors) and physically (baroreceptors). The first response depends on how much of and how long the cord is compressed. Complete compression causes the fetus to notice changes in blood flow and blood pressure, oxygen decrease, and carbon dioxide accumulation. The heart slows, and the blood pressure rises. Eventually, this changes to a decreasing heart rate and decreasing blood pressure. Chemical signals are released to modify this response until it is corrected. Usually, a one-time, one-minute, 100% compression of the cord takes five minutes to completely correct. But within that one minute, oxygen levels have decreased 50%, and the fetus must reset the valuable energy and chemistry it has expended. In a recent experiment, complete cord compression for five minutes required thirty minutes for recovery. Continued five-minute compressions every thirty minutes caused fetal decompensation. This happens because the fetus cannot reset all its hormonal, chemical, and nutrient baselines quickly. Some refueling takes longer to rebuild than others. The main fuel of the fetus is glucose. The fetus has its own store of crystalline glucose called glycogen in the liver, heart muscle, and elsewhere, but it does not use this emergency supply unless it is completely deprived of maternal glucose. This is important for its survival and proper cardiac function if stressed. When the fetus senses blood flow interruption, it also senses a variety of organ reactions. The liver reacts by changing blood flow to a vessel called the ductus venosus. This vessel also directly connects the fetal heart to umbilical blood flow, providing the fetus with more oxygen than is already available. The fetus shifts blood from its extremities to favor enough oxygen to its heart and brain. If the blood flow derangement persists after one minute, other systems join in to adjust for the loss of oxygen and nutrients. In addition to liver blood-flow changes, the fetus experiences blood shifts away from its intestinal blood supply and kidney blood supply. Renal (kidney) blood flow is altered, which, if sustained, will begin to change renal function. Adrenal glands responsible for releasing stress hormones now secrete cortisol, a stress steroid, and immediate-acting adrenaline called catecholamines. These chemicals alter the fetus's cardiovascular system (heart rate, blood pressure, pulse) and stimulate the fetus to adjust its position if related to cord compression. This positional change would be invoked by the fetus bending its thorax and neck and by inducing hiccups. All the fetal reflexes are now initiated and modified to achieve normal state. Once these events take place, the fetus is probably tired, like an athlete running a sprint, and it needs to recuperate. As the fetus rests, its urine changes composition and becomes more diluted, releasing Na+K+Cl ions.

Similar events probably take place in the fetal intestine; however, if the fetus used liver and heart glycogen, it cannot be replaced. If the glycogen store is low, it could create difficulty for the fetus if it continues to be stressed and is unable to depend on its only fuel storage. Heart dysfunction could eventually take place.

Fetal Behavior and Physiology Secondary to Cord Compression

In animal models, usually fetal sheep, repeated complete blockage of the umbilical cord changes the way the kidney excretes basic electrolytes. These molecules are important for basic-cell-function K+Na+Cl ions. If the cells of the body are unbalanced, they do not work properly. Improper cell functioning is similar to having a bad stomach virus with diarrhea and vomiting. In addition, this change is connected to the secretion of a hormone called vasopressin. Vasopressin is responsible for moderating blood pressure. When the fetus is stressed, it attempts to change its function until it relieves the stress. If cord compression is not relieved, further physiologic changes begin—the purpose of which is to conserve oxygen. Blood flow can be taken from the extremities (arms and legs) and other organs (such as the lung) and preferably shunted to the brain and heart. This preserves the brain and heart at the expense of the body and gives the fetus time (ten to fifteen minutes) to solve the problem of obstructed umbilical blood flow. If the fetus cannot correct the cord blockage, final changes begin to unfold. The fetus can tolerate these conditions as long as it has oxygen and glucose and it is not losing blood. But beyond fifteen minutes, the fetus begins to decompensate and experience tissue damage. The most vulnerable tissue is nervous tissue. As the brain loses oxygen, it turns to a backup nutrient called lactic acid. The problem with this brain food is that it does not metabolize cleanly and leaves buildup molecules called carbon dioxide; this situation causes the brain to swell, prompting blood vessels to close. Brain damage then occurs. The degree of damage depends on many factors, such as the age of the fetus at the time and the degree of oxygen loss to the tissues. As the lack of oxygen increases, the heart begins to fail. Not only does it malfunction in its role as a pump, but it also begins to short-circuit and develop arrhythmia, which is irregular heartbeats. These electrical-conduction defects put the fetus at risk for heart stoppage. If the fetus is low on oxygen (hypoxic), high on lactic acid and carbon dioxide (acidotic), and experiences heart arrhythmias, it will die. The fetus has behavioral patterns that can create cord compression and release. These reflex movements and organ adaptations have evolved over millions of years.

The overall relationship is a vigorous fetus having the ability to develop in the uterus without injuring itself, its cord, or its placenta while growing. The process of labor alters all these behaviors and recruits a new set of protective mechanisms designed to evade disruption of the supply line. During labor, compression patterns can change from a single short episode to repetitive cord compressions to prolonged compression where complete blockage forces immediate delivery. A typical example of complete blockage is a prolapsed cord where the cord enters the vagina before the fetal head. The cord can be compressed between the bony fetal head and bony maternal pelvis. Usually, fetal compromise will occur if delivery does not take place in ten minutes. A more detrimental accident is blood loss. Placental separation due to a short cord, umbilical cord rupture due to a defective cord, or a ruptured umbilical vein hematoma prompts not only blood loss but a lack of oxygen as well. These types of accidents can cause fetal death in minutes. Little can be done under these circumstances as these infants need immediate, rapid treatment with blood, fluids, oxygen, and support. If they survive, it is usually with damage. The animal model, which is not familiar to most, is the one that simulates intrauterine, prelabor, intermittent partial cord compression. This will be discussed in the next chapter.

> Management and treatment options for umbilical cord complications will follow an understanding of the basic pathophysiologic mechanisms. (Mann 1986)

> We rely greatly on information from animals; too much since there are great variations between species we know so little; measurements of flow of the umbilical (cord) are imprecise, and we have few measurements of human fetal arterial blood pressure, or of its changes with age.... Hence, much is speculative! (Dawes 1995)

Umbilical cord torsion untwisted (lower right)

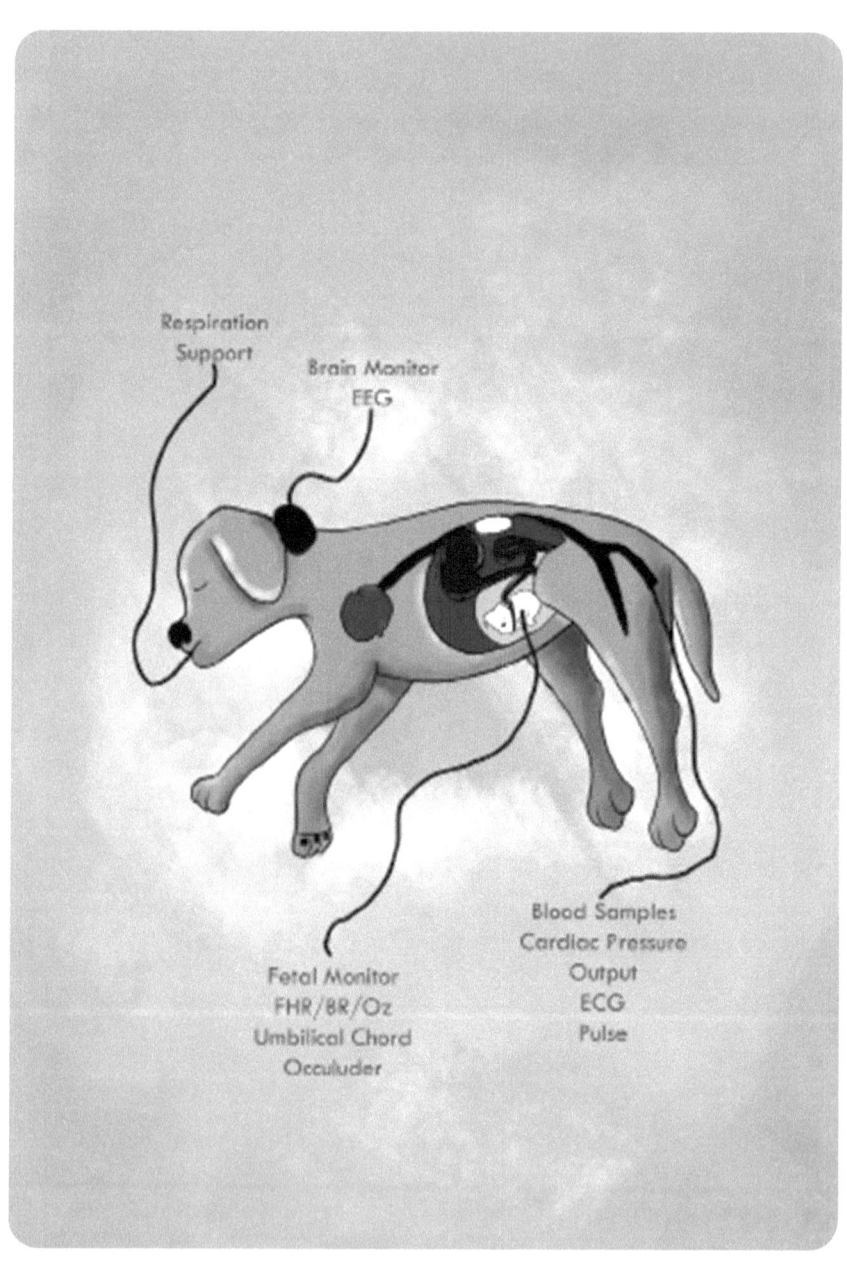

Animal Research

CHAPTER FOUR

What Animal Research Teaches Us about Umbilical Cord Accidents

> Animals will continue to be as vital as the scientists who study them in the battle to eliminate pain, suffering, and disease from our lives.
>
> —Heloisa Sabin speaking about
> Albert B. Sabin and polio vaccine research
> "Animal Research Saves Human Lives"
> *Wall Street Journal*, October 1995

Some of our knowledge about how the fetus behaves and is affected by supply-line disturbances comes from animal research. The ability to solve the problem of umbilical cord accidents may depend on future efforts involving research in animal models. From mice to rats to dogs to sheep to primates, valuable insights may only be possible using these heroes of research. Numerous dedicated world-class researchers depend upon animal models for their work. Many have contributed invaluable insights into how the fetus works. Translating animal-model research results to humans is not perfect and, at times, very different. Sometimes, too, human research gives insights to help animals. An important animal model for fetal physiologic research is the fetal sheep. This works out fairly well due to sheep tolerance of manipulation and similarity of human biology. Through sheep, scientists study fetal reaction to various forms of oxygen deprivation—one of the more poorly understood areas of obstetrics. Fetal sheep can be chronically oxygen depleted or acutely oxygen deprived, and the response to each situation differs. The time in gestational weeks and duration of a lack of oxygen in these models can be varied to show different fetal responses. There are several ways to study these events. One is to limit oxygen to the mother of the fetal sheep while the mother is under anesthesia. This, in turn, limits oxygen to the fetus. Another method is to limit blood flow to the uterus. Special techniques exist to reduce placental blood flow and simulate intrauterine growth retardation, which is thought to be due to similar conditions. Direct blockage of the umbilical cord can limit blood flow and oxygen delivery in varying degrees. These studies help scientists understand all the ways a fetus can be compromised. A specific animal model in sheep fetuses blocks the umbilical cord to simulate umbilical cord accidents. Several such studies have suggested insights into how supply-line interruption affects the heart, brain, kidneys, and metabolism of fetal sheep. When the umbilical cord is compressed in these models, characteristic fetal heart rate changes take place. One pattern type is called variable decelerations. Variable fetal heart rate decelerations are changes in heart beat-to-beat patterns that cause the heart rate to decline below normal levels (110 beats per minute). This is also a clinical sign used to determine whether a fetus needs immediate delivery. To understand how this works, fetal lambs had occluders placed around their umbilical cords while in the uterus. The occluders were opened and closed by timed pumps to simulate possible intrauterine events. Highly specialized, sophisticated equipment were used to measure the oxygen, acidity (pH), and other chemistries of fetal physiology. These studies showed fetal stress within the first thirty minutes of a two-hour experiment. The fetal heart rate reacted immediately, and the body chemistry changed quickly. Characteristic heart rate patterns called *W* signs, *U* signs, and *V* spike signs appeared. Fetal stress hormones began to rise and eventually became depressed or modified. In the sheep fetus, this suggests that time is an important factor when umbilical cord compression is occurring. Considering this on a human level, correction of cord compression over a reasonable amount of time is important. If the human fetal heart works like the sheep fetal heart, then neurological regulation of the fetus deteriorates with progressing acidemia and hypoxia caused by these compressions. Even if fetal death does not occur, the effects on the heart may be enough to permanently change the heart muscle. For example, a drop in fetal blood pressure creates a decrease in coronary blood flow and O2 delivery directly to the muscle. Indirectly, chemical products from the placenta abruptly enter the heart after release of cord compression. These, in turn, can affect the heart muscle with modified oxygen called oxygen free radicals. This excited molecule can burn heart muscle and change it. Vitamins such as C and E are called free radical quenchers. They can react with the excited oxygen molecule and return it to a normal state.

The chronically instrumented pregnant sheep and fetus have been used to study the effects of umbilical cord compression on neurologic function (figure 40). An overall view of complete cord compression showed an increasing tendency of the fetus to conserve blood flow between the heart and the brain, using oxygen from the limbs. This, in turn, directs oxygen to the more fragile neurologic tissue and away from the more durable gastrointestinal tract, muscle, and skeleton. This diversion appears to protect the brain and heart in that it buys time for a correction (see chapter Three).

These experiments give scientists a chance to look at the brain's reaction to cord compression. For example, depending on time, duration, and degree of blood flow interruption, various changes are seen. One change is edema (swelling) of the brain tissue. If severe, edema can be damaging. It is known that normal infants with uncomplicated births have edema for several days. How all this affects the fetus at different ages is unknown since animal models in mature sheep suggest that umbilical cord compression can cause varying types of damage with different insults of oxygen deprivation. Complete cord compression with complete loss of blood flow and oxygen may have several effects in term infants. In term sheep, these events cause hippocampal (learning center) damage after 10 to 15 minutes. Striatal (neuronal) damage occurs after repeated 5-minute compressions. This area contains white matter and is located lateral to the ventricles of the inner brain. Important cross connections to the brain's right and left hemispheres are located in the striatum. In different experiments, 50% blood flow interruption caused brain swelling, heart rate changes, and endocrine changes. Brain edema can press small blood vessels on the underside of the brain against the ridges of the skull and selectively reduce blood flow to specific areas. Heart rate changes can lead to arrhythmia of the heart and heart stoppage. When the cord is clamped and released over time in term sheep, other patterns of damage occur in the (white) brain matter. Similar patterns have also been observed in primates. In addition to neurologic changes, blood flow shifts from fetal organs and extremities to the placenta and heart are also documented (figure 41). These patterns are important to define if the mysteries of cerebral palsy and learning deficits are to be understood. During the 36th to 40th week of human gestation, significant damage appears to be possible due to combinations of hypotension, hypoxia, and stress caused by prolonged cord compression. While the fetal heart and brain are being protected during cord compression, the fetal adrenal gland is also being protected. The adrenal gland sits atop the kidney and provides stress hormones and chemicals. The adrenal gland usually reacts to danger in a fight-or-flight manner. For example, if stressed or compromised, the adrenal gland can turn on the launch signal prior to its due date. In the sheep fetus, when cord compression reduces blood flow, extremity (limb) circulation is shunted in part to the adrenal gland. This enhanced blood flow allows chemicals from the gland to be excreted to the fetus. The gland has two parts: an inside core and an outside capsule. The immediate response is to produce adrenaline (norepinephrine, epinephrine). These chemicals raise fetal blood pressure and stimulate the fetal heart to beat faster. In fetal rats, it may cause the fetus to jerk or move. While this occurs, the adrenal gland produces a stress hormone called cortisol, which protects the fetus from collapsing or having a nervous breakdown. These chemical signals go to the brain of the fetus that, in turn, sends signals to the mother that may ultimately cause release of oxytocin and, perhaps, vasopressin, all of which may initiate contractions.

The liver is another organ that may be stimulated during umbilical cord compression. An important fuel for fetal life that is stored in the liver is glucose. This is in crystalline form and presents in muscle and other tissues. One study examined glucose metabolism in fetal sheep and noticed increased glucose hormones (glucagon and insulin) during decreased O2 exposure. The placenta, cord, and muscle contain glycogen that, once used, is not restored. In chick and mouse fetal heart samples, the distribution of glycogen inside the cell changes with time. With maturity, glycogen increases in the cell structure called the mitochondria. This is the cell engine and provides energy for cell mechanisms. Muscle-cell glycogen stays about the same over time. The overall glycogen in the cell decreases from one day to thirty as if concentrated in the mitochondria. Only when the fetus turns to a postdelivery metabolism can it rebuild glycogen. This change in stored fuel may be important for other fetal conditions.

In addition, vessels in the liver tend to direct blood flow through an important vessel in one of several fetal shunts that are not needed after birth. Blood flow shunts are special vessels that redirect blood flow during fetal life. (Once born, these vessel detours are permanently closed to allow adult life.) Disturbances in these shunts may play a role in sending signals to the adrenal gland during stress through the right phrenic nerve. This nerve branch, which matures by twenty-four weeks' gestational age, could be an important emergency alarm that plays a role in quickly turning on stress chemicals when necessary. Umbilical cord compression also has direct effects on these shunts and their ability to stream blood to the heart.

Lungs are affected by these changes of blood flow through shunts in sheep animal models. Cord compression of 50% reduces lung interstitial blood flow. By altering O2 delivery, different patterns of damage are established. One of the effects of cord compression on lungs is the associate development of persistent pulmonary hypertension. This pathology has been demonstrated in a sheep model. A recent computer simulation model found that as the fetus shunts blood from the lower body to protect the brain and heart, lung oxygenation falls acutely. All current published facts point to a relationship between altered umbilical blood flow and lung maldevelopment.

Other lung effects unaddressed are fluid balance and surfactant production. The lungs are bathed in amniotic fluid, which participates in lung alveolar (air sacs) growth. It is unknown whether disturbances in water management can change the lungs' ability to mature. If the forty different lungs' cells are not receiving proper blood flow, they may not be producing chemistry to support lung functions such as O2/CO2 exchange. If fluid management is disturbed too much or there is too little fluid may alter how the fetus will breathe at birth. To date, no studies exist that consider amniotic fluid/lung function and relationships with chronic cord compression.

Thanks to expert studies of animal models, fetal responses to umbilical cord compression are known. A basic understanding of vital organs such as the brain, heart, kidney, lung, and adrenal gland will help determine how to help the stressed human fetus. The ability to study blood samples from both the mother and fetus will lead to methods to test the fetus and find the one needing delivery.

Some of the biochemical changes that can result from umbilical cord stimulation are as significant as organ, blood flow, and neurological changes. As the fetus experiences more stress, the tissues of the umbilical cord can secrete chemistry to react to the changes taking place. The local tissue reactions may be premature changes that would occur only during labor. Because the tissues cannot individually tell the difference, many false starts can take place. Local reactions in the umbilical cord by molecules released from the cells that line the umbilical vessels can cause momentary constriction or closure of the vessels. At birth, these molecules permanently close those vessels to prevent blood loss.

These small dynamic systems are constantly in balance. Thousands of these systems probably exist—some more immediate and more important than others. These systems are sometimes called autocrine and paracrine modulators, and they regulate local (cellular) chemical reactions. An obstetrical interest is the potential for a remedy to maintain blood flow. Discovery of a modulator that can be infused to the mother would be beneficial when there is evidence of blood vessel constriction. Animal-tissue studies can greatly enhance the understanding of these molecular effects. Studies in both human-tissue cultures and animal-tissue cultures have broadened our knowledge of umbilical cord-vessel endothelial cells. These are cells that coat the inside of umbilical arteries and veins. They produce the chemicals that respond to the conditions that occur moment to moment with the events of the placenta and fetal physiology.

LIST OF SOME PARACRINE/ENDOCRINE/AUTOCRINE MOLECULES

Oxygen—Several forms (modulators of other molecules)
Nitric Oxide—Relaxes placental vessels
Nitrite—Byproduct of oxygen and nitric oxide—inactive
Peroxynitrite—Byproduct of active oxygen—toxic to cells and active in the membrane of cells
Prostacyclin—Vasodilates placental vessels
Thromboxane—Constricts placental vessels and modulates coagulation
Endothelin-1—Constricts placental vessels
Epidermal Growth Factor—Tissue modulator
Poostanoids—Modulate coagulation of blood in umbilical vessels
Prostaglandins (PGE2)—Constrict umbilical vessels at birth
EGF + TGF—Constrict and regulate cord function
Xanthine/Purines/
Adenosine—Vasodilates placental vessels
Catecholamines—Stress molecules that modulate vessels
Nicotine—Vasoconstrictive
Caffeine—Unknown
Chocolate—Unknown
Herbal Tea—Unknown
Anesthetics-Bupivacaine—constriction of umbilical vessels
2-chloroprecaine—dilation of umbilical vessels

It is known that the amounts of these autacoids differ from umbilical vein to umbilical artery and from the placenta to the fetus. Anticoagulation autacoids (blood thinners) are higher in the umbilical vein; vasoconstrictor autacoids are concentrated toward the fetus, which means that they are important in stopping blood loss from the cord when it is severed. Epidermal growth factor, which makes PGE2, is located less on the placental end than the fetal end. This difference allows the constriction of cord vessels to begin at the placental end and peristalsis (squeeze) of blood toward the fetus. This trick of nature ensures an adequate blood count for the fetus. If this fails in large animals such as cows and horses, the newborn calf or foal will die of shock due to lack of blood volume.

Numerous regulators also exist outside and inside the umbilical cord. Amniotic fluid contains molecules from fetal metabolism, and blood circulating through the cord has molecules that are important to blood flow. It is amazing that any of us are born in one piece. These multiple systems can remain in balance and can adapt to disturbances. What is unknown is the limit of that adaptation. When does failure begin, and how long after failure does damage begin? Sometimes damage is immediate, sometimes it is confined, and sometimes it is chronic. To know these answers is to discover important ways to protect the fetus at risk. Animal models also allow research into other reproductive byproducts such as the placenta.

Determining the effects of fetal derangement on placental function is most important. Where the fetus can avoid injury, the placenta may not. No matter how vigorous the fetus is, it is in danger when the placenta deteriorates. The differences in placental structure from animal to animal allow varying effects. Sheep have multiple placentids where monkeys have one placenta like humans. Chimpanzees are better examples of human placental design.

Morbidity

Other Effects

Placental changes are important to study separate from fetal effects. These placental changes may or may not add to the fetus's ability to tolerate intermittent umbilical cord compression. The placenta has large reserves similar to other organs, where loss of placental tissue may be comparable to a loss of hearing in one ear, sight in one eye, or function of a kidney. The fetus can function and survive, but it may not grow and develop to 100% of its capacity. Cord compression may be a stimulus to induce such a compromise. It is theorized that if the umbilical blood flow is slowed, then placental blood flow is also slowed. When this happens, blood thickens in the small spaces in the placenta called the villous vessels and clots like gelatin. This, in turn, causes thromboses of the intervillous space that contains blood flow from the mother. The result is devitalized placental tissue and loss of that placental nutritional space. If enough dead space is developed, the fetus can be compromised. Thus, an indirect effect of cord pathology may be the secondary injury of the placenta even if the fetus does not, itself, become primarily injured. The umbilical cord complication observed that causes such a pattern is torsion (figures 42 and 43).

Animal placentas have been studied where torsion caused stillbirth of thoroughbreds (figure 44). Thrombi were seen in these placentas along with thrombosed surface vessels. Human placentas have been observed in cases of torsion where surface vessels were similarly thrombosed. The finding suggests multiple small blood-flow derangement episodes prior to death. Does this mean these events can be prenatally detected? It is possible that one day, ultrasound or maternal blood sampling will detect these changes. Another placental change that is more extensive than infarction of tissue is called chorangiosis. It is suggested that this change is due to low oxygen levels in the fetal circulation. This alteration of placental blood vessels looks like a rash. The vessels are dilated and full of blood cells. This change allows more surface area to grab more oxygen from the mother.

How much change is tolerated before fetal harm occurs is not clear. Chorangiosis and similar placenta changes have been studied in llamas and goats from high altitudes, especially in Chile. Because of low oxygen tensions at elevations above ten thousand feet, these animals provide an important insight into adaptations to tolerate chronic low-oxygen states. These changes seem to suggest that the chronically hypoxic (low oxygen level) fetus compensates with blood flow and blood cell expansion. To see similar changes in a fetus with cord entanglement suggests similar principles are involved.

All in all, multiple questions must be answered to solve the mysteries of umbilical cord compression. The answers may be forthcoming in each method of animal modeling used. Because of each unique characteristic of each species, study of the whole assemblage will be necessary to define umbilical cord-compression effects on the fetus.

RECOMMENDED READING

Gervaso F, Boschetti F, Pennati G. *Evaluation of the Wharton's jelly poroelastic parameters through compressive tests on placental and foetal ends of human umbilical cords.* J Mech Behav Biomed Mater. **2014** Jul;35:51-8.

Ferguson VL, Dodson RB. Bioengineering aspects of the umbilical cord. *Eur J Obstet Gynecol Reprod Biol.* 2009 May;144 Suppl 1:S108-13.

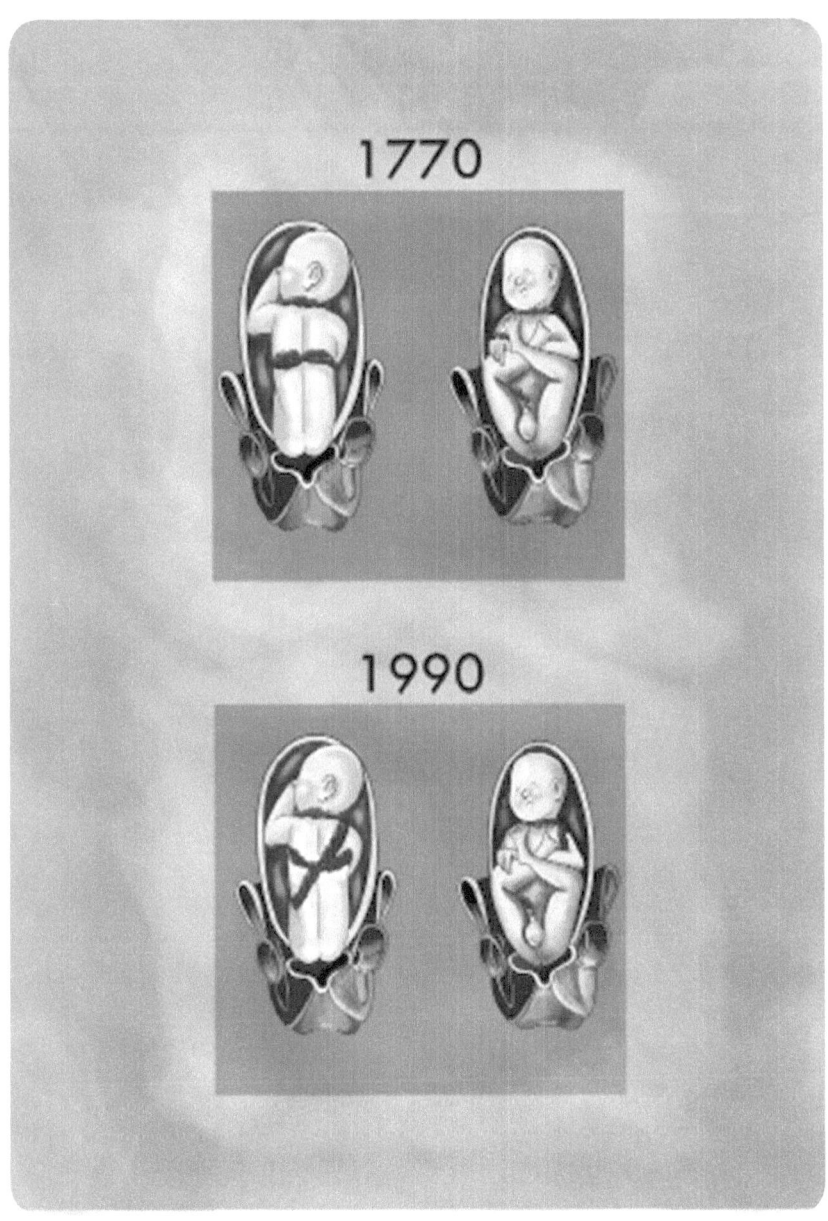

Umbilical Cord Entanglement

CHAPTER FIVE

Management of Umbilical Cord Anomalies, Abnormalities, and Complications

Fetal loss from umbilical cord abnormalities a difficult case for prevention.

—A. Ghosh, MD
Queen Mary Hospital
Hong Kong, 1984

"The baby who cheated death by 30 minutes: Doctors spot umbilical cord strangling foetus during routine scan and carry our emergency C-Section at 32 weeks."

http://www.dailymail.co.uk/news/article-2323349/The-baby-cheated-death-30-minutes-Doctors-spot-umbilical-cord...

Lucy LA,
Mail Online, May 12, 2013.

Managing the umbilical cord during pregnancy, labor, and delivery needs more discussion in obstetrical forums. In 1989, a publication from the US Department of Health and Human Services entitled *Caring for Our Future in the Content of Prenatal Care* describes specific pregnancy conditions or hazards. It comments that "structural abnormalities of the placenta are significant causes of poor pregnancy outcome." No other specific mention of umbilical cord-related events is listed, and no specific screening or management is suggested. This report of the Public Health Services Expert Panel on the Content of Prenatal Care did not address the issue of umbilical cord accidents but seemed to acknowledge an association with fetal harm. Increased discussions of cord-accident management are also important because this topic is virtually undeveloped and poorly defined. This fact is concerning because more infants are affected with cord complication than are with polio, AIDS, SIDS, pregnancy hypertension, gestational diabetes, or B-strep. The effects of umbilical cord-related complications can be as dramatic as a term stillbirth or as subtle as learning disabilities. It is consistent in that fetuses are being lost to cord accidents on a daily basis. The problem must not be understated. Once it was discovered that the polio virus caused harm, Dr. Salk was able to construct a management solution called polio vaccine. Umbilical cord accidents are causing stillbirth, asphyxia, emergency C-sections, fetal distress, and neurologic damage, which may consist of learning disabilities and cerebral palsy. How are these fetal harms to be prevented? Part of the difficulty in prevention seems to be in believing that an association exists. These relationships are difficult to demonstrate statistically. One analysis of cerebral palsy infants stated that looking at cord prolapse, body loops, and long cords, there were significant associations. All these insights are difficult to prove because the reviewed and relied-upon information is incomplete and full of statistical pitfalls. What can be done at this moment in time is to discuss and make clear the potentials of umbilical cord accidents. The attempt to manage cord problems during labor may go back to Zi-Ming Chen (AD 1237). His suggestion was to remove a shoulder loop by hand. "Doctor should ask the mother [to] lie on her back and be at rest, gently press its shoulder downward, and strip off the cord. Don't order the mother to exert her strength till the fetus positions itself properly."

In 1741, British obstetrician Dr. John Burton described several cases of cord management where delivery was impeded by a short cord and an entangled cord. "I was sent to a patient at Healey Manor who had been in labor about 30 hours . . . . I did imagine that the umbilical cord must be too short, and then I reached the string and found it fully stretched with the placenta strongly adhering to the womb. I therefore broke the string [cord] and delivered the woman . . . . I was sent to a person at Enwood . . . . I introduced my finger a little further and found the umbilical cord sat about the child's neck. I therefore twisted that part of the cord, which reached from the child's neck to the placenta, about my two forefingers and with my thumb broke it, withdrew my hand, when the child soon followed."

Dr. Nelson Sackett in 1933 described a case where he reached inside the uterus, encountered two loops around the baby's neck, and extracted the infant in the back position (version extraction), rupturing the cord in the process.

A study reviewing over one thousand births recently concluded: "From the point of avoidability of prenatal deaths, this study indicates that there is no clinical pattern and therefore no place of treatment for the obstetrician to save those babies which are killed by their own umbilical cord." (McLellan 1988)

This conclusion was based on traditional obstetrical care. There was no attempt to use tools such as ultrasound and fetal monitoring as a preventative measure. Some researchers have taken a different approach. In a case report of a stillborn with a nuchal cord × 2 and true knot, Dr. M. Maneschi (Universitad di Palermo, Sicily) in 1977 recommended that "a situation of this kind could be suspected on the basis of certain clinical findings to be elicited by questioning the patient about the intensity of active fetal movements, as well as in the presence of changes of position of the fetus and the findings of a high presenting part at term. If on the basis of these findings the cord is suspected to be short, either in itself or as a result of coils around the fetal neck or body and if low placental insertion and other causes of the high position of the presented part have been excluded by echography (ultrasound) further tests can be carried out."

Recently, Dr. N. V. Strizkova, chair of the Department of Obstetrics and Gynecology, Moscow Institute, and Dr. S. M. Petrikovsky, obstetrical professor, University of New York, used endoscopic devices in 1981 to visualize fetuses in the uterus with cord entanglement during labor.

Their solution was helpful in determining fetal risk once the membranes were ruptured. This attempt to manage the umbilical cord was followed by several scientific reports from China, Europe, Japan, and the United States, demonstrating ultrasound could visualize the umbilical cord.

Specifically, in 1982, P. Jouppila, MD (Oulu, Finland), described the ability to visualize the umbilical cord around the fetal neck. "Antepartum diagnosis of cord coilings would be of clinical value for the adequate suppression and management of this complication," he wrote. As ultrasound technology improved, more and more anecdotal reports appeared. Today it is recognized that ultrasound can visualize cord entanglement, abnormalities, hematomas, varices, knots, and architecture.

In a 1989 review by Dr. Ingo Clausen, professor of obstetrics and gynecology, University of Aarhus, Denmark, structural anomalies of the umbilical cord were mentioned as being diagnosed with ultrasound. Worldwide recognition that these potentially dangerous mechanical and acquired cord complications are responsible for antenatal fetal deaths is encouraging in that a solution and means of management are possible. Ultrasound visualization of cord position, structure, and function can be displayed in several forms. Black-and-white (grayscale) ultrasound can identify the outline (edges) of the cord and reveal the arteries and vein. Comparison to the fetus and placenta can detail both attachments and position. Doppler color ultrasound can visualize blood flow in color and outline the cord in red, blue, and yellow colors, depending on the direction of the blood flow. The two techniques provide a clear picture of cord condition relative to the fetus. The first step in managing the umbilical cord is visualizing it, and it can be visualized as soon as it forms. Measurements of the umbilical cord can begin as early as six to eight weeks. Knowing the length of the umbilical cord over time can help diagnose short or long cords and thereby anticipate difficulty with labor. Umbilical and placental insertion sites and characteristics can be visualized with ultrasonography. In addition, it is possible to visualize an abnormal placental insertion or an umbilical cord defect. The diagnoses of these cords have been described in many writings to date. Knowing that an abnormal insertion site exists may direct the obstetrician to look for growth disturbances.

In 1995, Dr. Torgrim Sørnes (Akershus Central Hospital, Norway) suggested that "there is an association between cord encirclement and fetal weight deviations, independent of cord length (effects)." An intense follow-up should be done on these fetuses. Another observation of cord abnormalities and fetal effects by Dr. John Rolschau (Odense, Denmark, 1978) states, "It has been documented that a thin umbilical cord is associated with low birth weight . . . Also, the RNA/DNA ratio was increased, indicating tissue stress (in the placenta) in cases of battledore insertions of the cord." Few studies have observed large numbers of infants from conception to delivery with these findings. This is necessary if the effects are to be accurately determined. A means of determining prenatally entangled fetuses having difficulty is needed. Case reports have been published on an individual basis where fetuses were prenatally observed with ultrasound and delivered when believed compromised. Torsion can be recognized by measuring the distance between the veins (pitch). A close pitch suggests multiple twists and the need to pay close attention to the fetus. Knowing which fetuses have the potential for umbilical cord complications is the next most important means of management is counting fetal movements. The mother can play an important role in preventing a tragic loss from a cord accident. While it is unknown how much time is needed for a fetus to die, it is believed that in most instances, the fetus dies slowly. As described earlier, fetal behavior is consistent, and if recognized by the mother, changes in fetal movement patterns can be documented and reported to the physician. Dr. E. Sadovsky studied movement among fetuses with cord complications and felt there was a pattern to signs of fetal stress. Older literature describes decreasing activity of the fetus over time. It is important for the mother to recognize when the fetus plays and when it sleeps. These activities should remain similar from thirty-two weeks until forty weeks. In addition, fetal strength should remain similar. However, fetal movement decreasing over time and weaker movement over time suggest fetal stress and should alert the mother to see her physician. Fetal jerking movement over time should also alert the mother. In addition, daily hiccup behavior (more than four episodes in twenty-four hours) suggests cord compression and initiation of fetal reflexes. These signs of probable fetal entanglement and/or placental insertion/location abnormalities should motivate the physician and mother to begin a surveillance plan, especially prior to forty weeks.

All detections of changes in fetal behavior noted by the mother or the physician should be shared with each other.

The second step is to measure (quantitate) fetal behavioral change. The simplest way is to evaluate the fetal heart rate, or FHR. FHR recordings of fifteen-minute strips can be invaluable during prenatal visits. Comparison over time can help identify a stressed fetus. The most sensitive indicator of fetal physiology is the heart rate pattern and characteristics. Fetal heart rate patterns change immediately with cord compression. Degree and duration of cord compression are unique. These patterns (called lambda signs, V shape, W shape, U shape, variable decelerations, late decelerations, and overshoot) indicate fetal blood flow disruption. Patterns that repeat themselves and develop frequently suggest a compromised fetus. These pregnancies can be identified and studied. One method is to evaluate the FHR at home at least once a week with a fetal monitor. This may allow the discovery of a slowly deteriorating pattern that indicates delivery. Potential delivery is suggested with the detection of a double nuchal cord, an abnormal FHR pattern at thirty-eight weeks, and a change in movement patterns for twenty-four hours.

It is well known that by thirty-six to thirty-eight weeks, the fetal colon is capable of peristalsis (movement) and contains bile acids for digestion, debris from swallowing vernix/lanugo, and cells. This intestinal mixture is called meconium. It is believed that the fetus expels this material, which discolors amniotic fluid to the well-known green color when motilin, an intestinal hormone, is released. The stimulus for the fetus to expel, or have a bowel movement, in the uterus is thought to be due to fetal stress. It is believed that one-fifth of all deliveries contain meconium. Whether or not this is correct, it is believed that the fetus is at risk under these circumstances. Meconium, whether thick or thin (diluted or concentrated), is damaging to fetal lungs if inhaled. It is also damaging to fetal membranes and can penetrate the membrane layers in one hour. If able to penetrate the amniotic barrier, cells called macrophages can transport these acids to the umbilical cord and can cause umbilical-vessel constriction. Experiments have demonstrated that umbilical arteries will be affected by meconium by stimulating the circular smooth muscle to tighten, thus closing the vessel off. This effect is observed to leave evidence of tissue damage as well as possible fetal circulation disturbances. Because meconium has the potential to lead to fetal compromise, it seems reasonable to avoid it. It is also possible that cord compression can cause the release of meconium by stimulating the release of motilin, creating additional cord-vessel constriction and blood flow interruption. This argues for close monitoring of fetuses with cord entanglement. The presence of meconium at birth does not mean or ensure that fetal damage has occurred. According to Dr. Naeye's study of the Collaborative Project, only 0.2% of the meconium-stained amniotic fluids examined were attributable to birth asphyxial disorders. However, Dr. Naeye stated: "After all of the antecedent risk factors had been taken into account, meconium in the amniotic fluid had only one unfavorable pregnancy outcome, the presence of neurological abnormalities at seven years of age. These neurologic abnormalities were of three types: quadriplegic cerebral palsy, lesser motor disorders with associated severe mental retardation, and chronic seizure disorders. These neurologic abnormalities are likely to be the consequence of vasoconstrictive effects of the meconium." A management goal, therefore, is to anticipate the fetus at risk and deliver it before a meconium accident. The timing may be difficult since it is believed that some fetuses can release meconium in small amounts and that it can be reabsorbed within twenty-four hours. There is debate about whether this is so, but it is known that the older the fetus, the more likely the occurrence. Fetuses are currently allowed to reach what is termed postmaturity. Yet fetuses older than a gestational age of forty-two weeks are considered postdates and are at risk of meconium. A management approach would be to consider any fetus with cord entanglement by its due date of forty weeks needs to be delivered. Doing so may avoid meconium in these infants as well as reducing stress factors to an already stressed state. In the Perinatal Umbilical Cord Project (PUCP), over one thousand fetuses have been screened, and no fetuses with obvious cord problems are delivered past forty weeks. None of these fetuses had meconium at delivery, suggesting that meconium is avoidable.

Ten percent of deliveries in the United States are associated with meconium. At least 1% have meconium complications. Fetuses prenatally diagnosed with umbilical cord complications should be aggressively managed to avoid meconium, and delivery should occur by forty weeks.

Unless this issue is proven unimportant by future scientific studies, assuming that meconium is not dangerous seems risky. To date, no such study has been done. Managing a fetus identified with an umbilical cord risk eventually requires a decision to deliver the baby. Reaching that decision can be difficult, especially where the fetus is early. Prior to the delivery date, a series of evaluations is necessary to document the physiological state of the fetus. The avoidance of a premature delivery is the concern of the obstetrician or caregiver. Collecting information on how to decide when to deliver a compromised fetus sometimes depends on information derived within the hospital. The fetus can be studied in more detail and its movements assessed with ultrasound. For example, its amniotic fluid can be measured to look for decreased urine output. If the fetus is not making urine, it could suggest it is weak and, therefore, ready to deliver even though it is not in labor. The fetus's blood pressure can be indirectly checked with color Doppler flow measurements. Its average heart rate and reactions to induced contractions (oxytocin stress test) can be assessed. If it is abnormal, delivery can be initiated. Tools are available to manage umbilical cord-related fetal changes. Ultrasound, fetal monitoring, and fetal movement counts are all now available to evaluate fetal health. Currently, no prenatal blood test can be simply performed. Some tests can remove blood from the fetus by amniocentesis and indicate if delivery is necessary. These tests are risky and may themselves cause labor and delivery. Two tests are interesting to discuss. One is called a blood gas; the other is called erythropoietin. A blood gas is an absolute measurement of the fetal well-being. The fetus's oxygen level, pH level, and related chemistries such as base excess can be quickly determined. A needle must be used to remove blood from the umbilical vein, requiring transabdominal/uterine penetration. If the blood shows acidosis (a low pH), it suggests the fetus is in need of delivery. A more recently developed test that measures fetal reaction to oxygen levels is erythropoietin, a hormone specific to red blood cell production. Preliminary tests suggest that an elevated erythropoietin level means the fetus needs oxygen and should be delivered if the level is sustained. Erythropoietin may also play a role in protecting neurologic tissue as it has been identified in the brain. Newborns with increased red blood cell production may show changes in the blood count test. Nucleated red blood cells appear as a result of the increased erythropoietin stimulus. These are immature cells, and many appearing on a test suggest a closer look at the fetus. None of these tests individually can decide whether a fetus should be prematurely removed from the uterus. Taken together, they form a solid base from which clinical judgment still must decide intervention based on experience. Management of newborns with cord-accident-related births goes beyond labor. Several tests are important to consider if a compromised fetus is delivered. A third step to consider is a premature infant that is showing signs of stress from an umbilical cord problem. Situations such as monoamniotic twins have been managed where betamethasone was administered by thirty-one weeks. This was done to mature the fetal lungs in the event of early delivery after thirty-two weeks. There are now several examples published where this was done. A case study of a single fetus with a double nuchal cord and true knot was managed this way and is presented at the end of this book.

Morbidity—Other Effects

> Nuchal-cord births have been observed to be predisposed to anemia. Not all nuchal-cord births are the same, but tight nuchal cords seem predisposed to producing anemia in the newborn. In one study, 18.5% of nuchal cords were anemic. The National Collaborative Perinatal Project defined perinatal anemia as a capillary hematocrit of less than 40% Hgb < 13.2 g/1 Hct < 39.1%. The information derived from this study suggests the need for hemoglobin and hematocrit determinations on all neonates who have nuchal cord [complications]. If symptomatic at delivery, hematologic evaluation should be done promptly and the neonate examined for evidence of hypovolemia and hypotension. If asymptomatic, hemoglobin and hematocrit determinations should be done before discharge from the nursery in order to identify those neonates who are anemic.
>
> Angela J. Shepherd
Department of Pediatrics
University of Texas, Galveston
AJDC Vol. 139, 1/1985 pg. 71

Nuchal-cord deliveries may also cause loss of fetal blood volume that, if greater than 20%, will induce hypovolemic shock. This is a condition where the fetus has lost too much blood. Observations have been reported where blood transfusions were necessary to correct this emergency. The clinical picture is different from lack of oxygen in that blood volume is missing but oxygen levels are normal. The newborn is usually characteristically pale, tachycardiac with irregular respirations, and weak with a low blood pressure. This physiologic state is caused by decreased perfusion of tissue rather than an absence of oxygen and nutrients. The metabolic activity of the tissues remains static, so the chemical activity has nowhere to go—like a stagnant pond. Byproducts, therefore, have no place to go, and oxygen, although available, cannot enter the cell. The result is a buildup of waste products and carbon dioxide that results in cellular acidosis. This dangerous state can cause death if not corrected. Once discovered, hypovolemia is quickly treated with fluids, plasma, and blood transfusion. These events are not common but do happen. Indeed, knowing that the potential for morbidity exists can be enough to quickly recognize this clinical emergency. Newborns with cord problems should be reviewed for morbidity. Blood also contains cells that react to tissue damage called white blood cells (WBC). Many types of white blood cells are called by various names, depending on the cell purpose. A polymorphonuclear leukocyte (WBC/PMN) is a cell very important in protecting tissues from bacteria and other invaders. It is also important in reacting to tissue that has been damaged by changes in blood flow. Tissues that line blood vessels such as umbilical arteries and veins are called endothelial cells and, under high microscopic magnification, look like ceramic tiles. These cells contain chemicals that, when released, can react with PMNs and incur damage. These reactions over time can affect the smaller vessels of the placenta or elsewhere and eventually contribute to organ dysfunction. Not only does the fetus react as a whole to cord compression and as a biologic agent on a cellular level, but it also reacts on a molecular level. A rapidly emerging field in the medical sciences is one of molecular research. It is the step up from genetics and the step below cellular activity, but all are interrelated.

A possible marker for tissue damage is another WBC called a lymphocyte. Recent research by Dr. Naeye suggests that compromised fetuses that develop neurologic injury enough to cause cerebral palsy have changes in their lymphocyte counts. When reviewing records of a group of CP infants, lymphocyte counts of greater than ten thousand were noted. These elevations did not occur in any less severe circumstances and did not recur. The changes seem important in determining when neurologic injury took place. The timing of stillbirth will be discussed based on the appearance of the infant. These concepts of forensic studies are important if scientists are going to understand how umbilical cord accidents affect the fetus over time. With more multidimensional genetic markers and factors being uncovered, a better understanding of fetal death will emerge. What lies in the future is speculative, but now a solution is possible.

How Will Future Umbilical Cord-Complicated Pregnancies Be Managed?

The initial step is to visualize the baby. Mothers who have experienced a stillbirth should be studied with multiple ultrasounds during the subsequent pregnancy. Why? At the very least—to put them at ease. There is no unnecessary ultrasound in this group of patients. Very soon, 3-D printers will be able to translate the image into a physical product that can be held by the mother.

Nonstress test: "Our results suggest that the non-stress test should be used as the primary test for antepartum detection of fetal acidosis because it has the highest sensitivity; in addition, it is simple and easy to perform." (Vintzileos 1991)

Managing UCA

CHAPTER SIX

The Future of Umbilical Cord Research

The goals of prenatal research must be to prevent cerebral palsy, to improve our understanding of prematurity, to give every baby its right to a sound body and mind when she or he is born, and perhaps one day make the NICU as obsolete as the iron lung [for polio].
—Peter W. Nathanielsz, MD, PhD, ScD
Ithaca, New York 1995

Where there is no vision, the people perish.
—Proverbs 29:18a KJV

What can be expected in the future of research into umbilical cord complications? To conduct the research, resources must be obtained to pay for the sophisticated technologies and supplies needed. Trained personnel such as nurse-midwives, medical statisticians, obstetricians, pathologists, and engineers will be needed, as well as competitive salaries. A review by the Institute of Medicine published in 1992 states that obstetrics and gynecology lack supporters in government research agencies. In its survey, it is estimated that six to eight physicians/scientists each year are recipients of major training support. Only 9 out of 250 departments of obstetrics and gynecology nationally received more than $2 million in federal funds in 1990. On one federal advisory committee, it was noted that there was a scarcity of obstetrics and gynecology representation even though a major source of hospital admissions to most acute-care hospitals is from ob/gyn. Overall, the share of research funds from federal sources going to departments of obstetrics and gynecology has remained at a steady 1.5%. Given adequate funding, the solution to umbilical cord complications is reachable. It appears possible that one solution to cord entanglement is to reach into the uterus and reverse it.

Today, Dr. Michael Harrison at the University of California, San Francisco, enters the uterus as early as twenty-four weeks' gestational age to repair holes in fetal diaphragms. This deadly defect, which occurs in about 1 of every 2,200 births, has been successfully treated this way.

Surgical manipulation of the uterus and fetus is highly complex and very risky. The demonstration that it can be done is equivalent to the Wright Brothers' first flight. The steps necessary to surgically repair diaphragmatic hernias are more involved than the steps it would take to untangle a fetus identified at risk, an event that may be many times more common than 1/2,200 for diaphragmatic hernia or 1/600 for mongolism risk. Every umbilical cord abnormality places the fetus at risk for stillbirth. This may be a 1/500 risk. Fetal harm without stillbirth may be 1/50 risk and unrecognized. Entering the uterus with an endoscope smaller than the diameter of a pencil is possible. By comparison to a uterine incision, the endoscope is significantly smaller. It essentially avoids trauma. Over the last decade, this experiment has been performed in animals and humans with success. This suggests that a fetus imaged with 3-D ultrasound and diagnosed with entanglement at twenty-four weeks can be identified. Fetal heart rate changes compatible with cord compression can be visually evaluated and a fetus at risk for complications followed. Today, needles are used to sample the umbilical cord for blood in infants with stress and illnesses. These invasive procedures are successful and proven to save fetuses' lives. A hook wire is inserted into the uterus to manipulate the cord. Several recent reports have used small-gauge devices to manipulate the cord, puncture it, and suture it. One report described the use of this technique to obstruct the cord of a dead twin who was taking blood flow from a live twin. All these efforts taken together say that entering the uterus with several small-diameter devices to visualize the fetus, identify the cord, remove the entanglement, and leave the fetus to heal and grow in the uterus is possible today. Reports from the Netherlands have demonstrated successful visualization of the fetus with an endoscope in monkeys, which does not disturb the mother or create premature labor. To accomplish the goal of fetal surgery for cord entanglement, funds are needed to design the equipment and to work with an established animal-model laboratory with trained technicians and certification. To purchase a research monkey for study and its necessary support costs at least $2,000 per monkey. This type of research is absolutely necessary to demonstrate to governmental authorities such as the Food and Drug Administration that these surgical techniques are safe and effective and can avoid stillbirth. Without this documentation, approval of these techniques will not take place.

Another approach being evaluated by the Pregnancy Institute uses fetal heart rate monitoring. Currently being studied is a surveillance approach that depends on telemetry (remote telephone monitoring). Selected patients with cord-entangled fetuses are equipped with special monitors at home. These home fetal heart rate monitors are used by the mother to record fetal heart rate strips for telephone transmission. At prescheduled times, the monitoring episodes are watched in real time by the physician at home. This allows the patient to be home and allows the physician to choose a convenient time. Surveillance with telemetry-based fetal heart rate monitoring is done every night until delivery, usually thirty-six to forty weeks. It has been done as early as twenty-eight weeks for two months straight. This clinical trial, as of this writing, has home monitored over one hundred patients with previous loss due to UCA. These patients are located across the United States and overseas.

> Stillbirth In non-malformed babies of birth weight greater than or equal to 2.51 kg. these babies are apparently well equipped to survive until the terminal event [normal but dead] and on the basis of this study there is likely to be a high degree of avoidability to their deaths. (Kirkup 1990)

Statistical understanding of umbilical cord-related stillbirths is inaccurate at best. Future efforts to more accurately depict events leading to stillbirth are needed. Publications from New Delhi, Norway, China, Scotland, Germany, Britain, and the United States cannot accurately determine how many antenatal or neonatal deaths are due to the umbilical cord. Because of inaccurate reporting by death certificates state by state, the National Center for Health Statistics cannot determine the extent of this mortality. Fetal harm (morbidity) is completely unknown and unavailable. One Chinese study suggested morbidity consisted of neurologic damage and neonatal deaths. What worldwide statistics exists is largely based on labor and delivery events and not prenatal events. One study reviewed perinatal deaths in normal infants and related lack of antenatal care by twenty weeks as an important risk factor. In 30% of deaths, there was an avoidable factor. In 61% of these cases, intrapartum management appeared to be an important factor. The most important aspect of management was recognition of fetal heart rate monitoring abnormalities.

In *Life* magazine, July 1969, Dr. Edward Hon is shown reading a fetal heart rate pattern recording from a fetal monitor he invented. The recording showed repeat fetal heart decelerations. An image of the delivered infant (breech delivery) was shown with of a single tight nuchal cord.

> Abnormal Fetal Heart Rate Patterns may be present for many minutes before actual fetal death. Changes in fetal heart rates associated with umbilical cord compression may be progressive over many minutes and hence useful . . . . Therefore, many of the avoidable factors detected related to the recognition of probable fetal distress by fetal heart rate monitoring these heart rate abnormalities arose 3 hours before death and did not resolve or remit but went unattended. (Hon 1975)

Estimating the time of death in stillborns is important in order to understand factors causing death. What events lead to the death of a fetus especially when the supply line is involved? In normal no-risk (no illness) pregnancies, this insight would be invaluable.

> A large review of cord related stillbirths needs to be done to determine the timing of death. Is it random, circadian, nightly,

daily during maternal activity, rest, after meals, etc.? Here again there had been recognition of life within 4 days of delivery indicating that the fatal compression occurred with the advent of labor.... The mother had been uneasy about diminished foetal movements although the foetal heart was still distinctly heard; then within 2 days, the foetal heart disappeared. (Corkill 1961)

Some insights about the timing of death may be discoloration of the umbilical stump; desquamation (loss of skin) of the face, abdomen, or back; brown skin discoloration; and mummification. These changes correspond to six, twelve, twenty-four hours or to great changes from death to delivery. Reviewing stillbirths for these changes may help pinpoint time of death and fetal symptoms perceived by the mother.

Numerous examples have been published describing isolated case reports of maternal symptoms related to the cord mechanism involved. Reports include statements such as pulling sensations from the cord insertion site to great movements of the fetus as it changes position, or a stick on a picket fence, as the abdomen of the mother is stimulated with fetal repositioning. Fetal jerking movements and hiccups are not uncommon complaints with nuchal cords and knots. Rolling movements are detected by the mother. Even seizures have been described. The most important symptom is decreased fetal movement, sometimes days before death. We continue to tell patients that the fetus should not slow down toward term. The mother needs to be aware of fetal behavior. Patients can feel what the fetus is telling them. Every symptom and subtle sign should be used to suspect fetal compromise.

In European countries, intrauterine fetal death (IUFD) is responsible for more than half of the perinatal mortality rate. The intrauterine fetal death rate reflects the complete failure of pregnancy surveillance and antenatal care. Therefore, the development of specific strategies in order to further reduce stillbirths becomes more and more important. More than one-third of stillbirths reported in Europe seemed predictable and avoidable by appropriate management after a positive fetal surveillance test. More than 50% of the stillbirths occurred after the thirty-fourth week of gestation, when any infant has a nearly 100% chance to survive with modern pediatric care. At the same time, a marked decrease in the number of antenatal visits and quality of antenatal surveillance can be observed in cases of antepartum stillbirth. It should be concluded that antenatal surveillance has to be performed more intensively, especially in the last trimester.

> Intrauterine fetal death is the worst result of antenatal care for the obstetrician and creates tremendous grief with parents in the knowledge that they have lost an infant with full potentials for later life. (Scheider 1994)

Two types of deaths seem to be related to cord complications: sudden death, such as with cord rupture, hematoma, prolapse, and maybe entanglement; and slow death, such as with nuchal cords, knots, torsion, and body loops. There are early deaths and late deaths, which may have different patterns.

Management of patients facing this potential harm will require different strategies. Noninvasive approaches will use ultrasonography to discern the fetus at risk. Future evolution of techniques using chemical factors from the maternal blood may be useful in following that specific fetus. Detecting fetal chemical changes from the maternal blood sample may allow the evaluation of a slowly dying fetus and the decision to intervene with delivery if late or to intervene with manipulation of the fetus if early.

One older manipulation is external version. With computer assistance, knowing that the nuchal cord is entangled right to left, the fetus might be manipulated to unwind the loop. This is done by using one's hands on the pregnant abdomen and maneuvering the fetus around head to toe. These potential management techniques will have to be tried to determine their feasibility. To imagine this maneuver, compare it to the game of 3-D movements inside a round frame. Like the game, the procedure could be used to slowly rotate the mother to induce countermovements in the fetus, thus untangling it. Although this may seem far-fetched, with computer guidance and imaging, it may be possible. Another possible insight may be derived from NASA's Ames Research Center. NASA and specialists from the University of San Francisco's Fetal Treatment Center are developing devices that would be placed inside the uterus with the fetus. These devices would measure fetal vital signs. The intrauterine space becomes a tailored NICU. The biotransmitters send vital information by radio signal to be evaluated by computers outside the fetus. Already in existence is a thermometer capsule that is swallowed by astronauts to measure core body temperature. NASA codeveloped this capsule that sends constant temperature readings to a monitor by radio signal. The ability to continuously know fetal blood pressure, heart rate, EKG patterns, and oxygen/pH status will be important. Ultimately, it will be necessary to know glucose/lactic acid/catecholamine/erythropoietin and cortisol/ACTH levels. These chemistries provide insights into the fetal condition and would assist in deciding the need for delivery. For instance, a cord-entangled fetus with decreased movement, low oxygen levels, and elevated erythropoietin might need delivery. Current fetal blood tests attempting to determine time of injury only determine damage already done. These tests include measuring fetal lymphocyte counts over time. In the future, it may be possible to detect early changes as the damage is beginning and rescue the fetus before irreparable harm occurs.

Umbilical cord complications can be solved just as polio was solved. It is important to do so because the fetuses are normal. They are not defective, malformed, or irreparably injured. What is required is support to create the solutions. The solutions are at hand.

> At present, we can offer no single solution to the problem of umbilical cord complications which remains probably the most important cause of fetal depression at birth. (Bruce 1978)

> By means of a model similar to that of Clapp, et al we have reported evidence of an increase in free oxygen radicals as possible causal factor in cerebral lesion. These observations [of umbilical cord compression/blood flow reduction] should alert physicians to pursue more investigative studies on the potentially ominous FHR pattern in relation to the long term outcome of the infants, particularly that of neurologic performance. (Murata and Quilligan 1994)

Umbilical Cord Genetics:

http://discovery.lifemapsc.com/in-vivo-development/umbilical-cord.
Gene sets have been described in umbilical cord tissue, mainly in mesenchyme stem cells. It is unknown what chromosome is or are involved in umbilical cord development and properties. DNA has been extracted from umbilical cord tissue. RNA has been more difficult to extract and identify especially in stillborns. New methods of genomic identification are emerging constantly.

Stillborns may have specific profiles and markers which could determine cause of death. One such marker is the Hypoxic Inducible Factor HIF1. Future studies might be able to distinguish a cause of death which is oxygen related or other cause based on HIF1. Levels of stress or hypoxia can trigger specific gene expression the profiles of which may be helpful in a stillbirth investigation. There may be marker evidence in organs sensitive to hypoxia such as the kidney and heart a profile of which may point to other mechanisms of death. The heart has a marker called Troponin which identifies specifically heart muscle injury. It is a test used frequently in cardiology. This marker has been reported in newborns with asphyxia at birth. Micro heart damage has been described in these babies.

Umbilical cord gene expression has been shown to predict premature babies at risk for lung disorders. Other investigations have shown effects of maternal smoking. Gene expression translates into biochemical pathways which can be identified as different in stillborns vs liveborns. Eventually these genetic advances will clarify cause of death.

Cord compression may rapidly influence the expression of placental angiogenic genes in pre-eclampsia. *Järvenpää J, Vuoristo JT, Ukkola O, Hirvikoski P, Savolainen ER, Raudaskoski T, Ryynänen M. Placenta. 2008 May;29(5):436-8. doi: 10.1016/j.placenta.2008.02.010.*

Case Studies

(I) A Difficult Case for Prevention
A Combination Umbilical Cord Accident

This term pregnancy in a twenty-eight-year-old G3 P1 AB1 was uneventful until one weekend before the due date. Fetal movement ceased after a day-long fishing trip. Evaluation on labor and delivery indicated a fetal demise. Spontaneous vaginal delivery revealed a stillborn male fetus ($7\frac{1}{2}$ lb) with three nuchal cords, a shoulder loop-body loop, a two-vessel cord, straight architecture, and a true knot. In addition to these findings was a cord length of 100 cm and marginal placental insertion. Which abnormality caused death is disputed in the medical literature. When and how these fetuses die are difficult to document. Whether diet plays a role or maternal activity changes uterine physiology are unclear. The Perinatal Umbilical Cord Project (PUCP) seeks to address the problem of umbilical cord accidents.

(II) Time of Death:
Nuchal Cord Type B and Clinical Clues

A thirty-year-old white female G1 P0 was doing well prenatally up until twenty-eight weeks when the fetus was noted to be breech turned from vertex. A single nuchal cord was diagnosed, and fetal heart rate changes were in normal range. Reexam at thirty weeks confirmed a breech lie with a NCX1 and normal FHR. A scheduled return in two weeks and expected repositioning of the fetus to vertex was preempted by stillbirth two days before the revisit. Saturday night, the patient noted fetal movement of normal strength and duration at 10:00 p.m. The fetus was breech and did not exhibit jerking movements or hiccups, suggesting no stress during the breech lie. Awakening at 7:00 a.m. on Monday morning, no movement was felt as expected. An office visit confirmed fetal demise, and an ultrasound showed a triple nuchal cord and a vertex lie. At delivery, a normal male (6 lb) had a triple NCX3 with a type B NCX1 (see text). Also seen was a marginal cord insertion into the placenta. Microscopic exam of the placenta showed chorangiosis (a placental change associated with asphyxia). The Perinatal Umbilical

Cord Project (PUCP) has observed there are two types of nuchal cords (A and B) and that these stillbirths may occur at night during sleep.

(III) Fetal Heart Rate Changes:
Warning Signs of Cord Compression

Over one thousand pregnancy cases and counting have been reviewed for cord complications in the Perinatal Umbilical Cord Project. What has repeated itself over and over are the fetal heart rate patterns associated with cord compression. Depending on the degree of compression, duration, intermittency, and gestational age of the fetus, fetal heart rate responses tell us a lot about this event prior to labor. Three cases briefly described here suggest a variety of presentations.

Case KD
A thirty-year-old G3 P2 with normal deliveries previously. This fetus developed a shoulder loop and fetal heart rate changes prior to labor. Subsequent resolution of the shoulder loop occurred during a next-day OCT. Delivery was uneventful, but the newborn had a persistent ductus arteriosus, and the placental exam showed choragiosis, a pathology of placental stress. At five years old, the young girl is developing normally.

Case TR
A thirty-five-year-old G4 P3 developed an arrhythmia during labor. An intermittent arrhythmia was noticed prenatally. As labor progressed, the arrhythmia became more pronounced. Eventually the FHR became nonreassuring, causing a C-section. A posterior placenta with marginal/sacral umbilical insertion was present. The newborn EKG was abnormal for two hours. Cause unknown.

Case MB
A twenty-seven-year-old G1 P0 at term with a prenatally diagnosed nuchal cord X1 progressed to 6 cm, +1 station when sudden bradycardia developed. An emergency C-section was necessary to relieve the umbilical cord compression and developing metabolic acidosis. Note the developing arrhythmia and increasing frequency prior to delivery. A similar physiology may be the event occurring prenatally that leads to stillbirth of similar cases.

(IV) Umbilical Cord Risk Managed After a Previous Cord Accident

Case MS

A twenty-seven-year-old G2 P0 SB1 had a previous stillbirth associated with a double nuchal cord. Her subsequent pregnancy was monitored with frequent ultrasounds and FHR monitoring. At twenty-eight weeks, a double nuchal cord was seen on ultrasound. At thirty-two weeks, a true knot was verified. Delivery by thirty-six weeks confirmed a double nuchal cord with true knot. The patient correctly recognized decreased fetal movement and changes in the fetal heart rate (on home monitoring).

(IV) Umbilical Cord Risk Managed After a Previous Cord Accident with Subsequent Morbidity TF

A twenty-eight-year-old G3 P1 SB1 was being monitored for repeat cord risk. Her previous stillbirth was due to a double nuchal cord and triple knot at thirty-six weeks. During the third pregnancy, a nuchal cord was diagnosed by thirty-two weeks and followed to thirty-six weeks, where decreased fetal movement and fetal heart rate variables prompted delivery. At forty-eight hours, the infant developed persistent pulmonary hypertension and required NICU care and oscillator support for one week. At six months, the newborn was well. Cord compression may be associated with pulmonary hypoxia due to shunts delivering blood flow to the adrenal gland, heart, and brain. Animal-model studies have suggested this connection. Recent computer cord-blood-flow models also suggest loss of pulmonary blood flow during fetal stress, hypotension, and low cord flow. Pulmonary injury may not be uncommon.

(VI) Umbilical Cord Torsion, a Not Uncommon Occurrence in Newborns

Umbilical cord torsion is usually not diagnosed in a live born. Ten percent of deliveries may have uncomplicated torsion. Torsion can coexist with constriction, a different pathology altogether. Amniotic bands may also be present with both the former pathologies. *No* published stillbirth study has included umbilical cord torsion in its database, which brings the results into question.

The following publication describes two cases of repeat UCA in the same mom. The explanation is that the fetal reflexes that lead to entanglement can recur under the same reproductive conditions. Patients have reported as many as four to five births each with nuchal cord, knots, and torsion. UCA events are not rare; they can repeat in the same mom and family (such as long cords) and can repeat similar developmental characteristics.

Multiple tight coils of funis with repeated fetal death.

by MM. H. Vermelin and J. Richon
"Multiples circulaires serrés avec mort foetale"
Société d'obstétrique et de gynécoogie de Nancy
1950
(Traduced from French by Laura Adam)
10/15/2009

Multiples tight coils of funis with repeated fetal deaths
Let us describe you two observations:

Observation 1.—Ms. A . . ., 29 years old, mother of two daughters aged of 10 and 2 years old, became pregnant in January 1950. She was supposed to give birth by the end of October.
    The 10th of October, she feels the first contractions and enters in the maternity hospital. After a rapid 3 hours labor, she ejects a 3.400 kg boy. His head is freeing up with difficulties and remains locked at the vulva. We hardly lower the occiput and notice that there exists, at the neck emplacement, three tight coils of funis, so tight that the umbilical cord has a reduced volume, forming a real whitish lace. After rapidly cutting the cord, we notice that the baby's neck is cut by the coils and that the skin is snatched at certain sites. The child hasn't any heart beats anymore: he is pale and cannot be resuscitated. The cord's length was 44 cm. This woman gets pregnant two years after. The childbirth was planned for the last days of June. The 1st of July, when she enters in the maternity hospital, the head is high but applies conformably to the

[DS???]. The cervix is dilated to 3 cm. Two hours later, the dilatation is complete. The head is at the medium part. Because of the previous incidents, we check very regularly the fetal heart after each contraction. Foetus heart beats are goods. As soon as the urge to eject the baby arrives, beats remain very slow after each contraction and we decide to finish with an application of forceps in [GT ???], at the medium part of the excavation. With some difficulties, we bring the head at the lower part, and as in the first case, the enucleation of the head is difficult: we notice with astonishment, four coils of funis very tight, binding the neck of the foetus, that we promptly cut. We extract the baby: a 3.400 kg boy without any heart beat. The cord measured 50 cm.

Observation 2.—Ms. S . . . is 29 years old in 1951.

She gave birth in 1947 in the maternity hospital, in 1949 at home, and in 1951 at Charleville, two boys and a girl that grew up normally.

The 30th of April 1954, she delivers a 3.800 kg boy at home; he presents the start of a fetus sanguinolentus and has one very tight coil of funis.

Her fifth delivery takes place the 1st of March, 1956. At noon, when she enters at the maternity hospital, the dilatation was 4 cm—the amniotic sac was intact—fetal beats were irregular and muffled.

At 5pm, spontaneous split of the pouch: mushy pea liquid. The head was at the high part of the excavation in [G.P. ??]. Beats not sensed.

At 7pm, complete dilatation and ejection of a boy weighting 3.600kg in 10 minutes. There exists one tight coil that we cut using pliers. The baby is flabby but presents some heartbeats.

The baby dies in [word absolutely unknown, it sounds like "slightly raised from death"], a few minutes after, despite the usual cares.

If we look at the death toll of this sinister series of foetus deaths, one recent foetus sanguinolentus and three fetal death at ejection, we can only notice the presence of the danger of coiling of funis.

This danger is a constant threat and the fact that it is unpredictable makes it more serious.

At present, there is no investigation method to asses or declare null the existence of coils in the cord. Even if one day we can predict, before delivery, the presence of one or more coils, how many children are born with loose coils.

Too many considerations are involved: length of the cord, thickness of the cord, movement of the foetus, repetitive careful attempts of [version??] by external operations, which each of them or all of them, can create one or more coils.

The late engagement to the presentation due to the fact that the foetus is trussed by a short cord is not a possible criterion for tight coils above all for the multiparous.

The only solution for the obstetrician is to check the quality of the foetus heart beats, far from being an absolute solution. How many times beats are slowly and affected for a while during the ejection.

Proceeding to an emergency Caesarean section when we know there were previously a mortal foetal accident can appears as a legitimate advise, in condition that this caesarean is wittingly made, for an healthy foetus and not for a dying foetus on which anoxia would have already causes irreversible encephalo-meningal [???] lesions. And how many useless sections will be practice in those cases! At present, it seems that obstetrical trauma, cause of the fetal death by funic compression (cord prolapses and coils of funis) represent 1% of neonatal deaths. Canon, Guillem and Mayer evaluated in 1953 to 9% the risk of neonatal anoxia purely due to funic.

Anoxia caused by funic remains a heavy mortgage weighting on delivery and which doesn't seem to be definitively removed presently.

A recent e-mail tells the same story of repeat loss due to UCA.

> **From:** Erica
> **To:** haydel1@bellsouth.net;
> **Date:** Tue, January 15, 2008 11:13:48 PM
> **Cc:**
>
> **Subject:** Dr. Collins, I have had two stillborn babies Dr. Collins, I am 27 years old. I read about you online and the research you are doing on stillborn babies. My first baby was stillborn at almost 35 weeks in August of 2006 and I recently lost my second baby at 30 weeks on December 18, 2007. We have no answers as to why this has happened twice. The doctors see nothing wrong with the cord, placenta, etc. Both baby girls have been born looking perfectly healthy and the first autopsy revealed nothing, we are still waiting on results for our 2nd baby's autopsy. I believe that

they both passed away in the middle of the night because I felt each of them moving before I went to sleep and felt no movement the next day. My husband and I desperately want a healthy baby and are devestated that this nightmare has happened twice.

I appreciate your time.
Erica

Umbilical cord accidents can repeat in the same patient (mother). They can be identified with ultrasound, managed with fetal heart rate monitoring, and successfully delivered. No baby should be stillborn after thirty-six weeks due to a UCA. The solution requires intensive observation and identification of the fetus at risk for this silent complication.

Ethics of Reporting test results to patients:

The American Medical Association publishes a text *Code of Medical Ethics*. In the edition for 2008-2009 pg 259 "Reporting Clinical Tests: General Guidelines" it states ;"Any information gathered from test results that would be necessary for patients to make intelligent medical decisions and give informed consent on future medical treatment must be disclosed to them"

The following protocol can help prevent UCA.

Protect your Pregnancy-Pregnancy Institute Protocol

Ultrasound Can Visualize the Umbilical Cord

- 10-12 weeks: a vaginal ultrasound to measure the crown-to-rump length of the baby.

- 18-20 weeks: anatomical description of the umbilical cord and its placental and fetal connections.

- 26-28 weeks: umbilical cord review documenting its position and characteristics.

30-32 weeks: umbilical cord review documenting its position and characteristics.

36-37 weeks: umbilical cord review noting the presence of cord entanglement, twisting, compression location near the rump or baby's head.

If an ultrasound review documents a finding, more frequent prenatal visits are needed. After twenty-six weeks, the baby has a good chance of survival if delivered early. If entanglement is noted on an ultrasound study, weekly ultrasounds will be needed. Fetal heart rate testing twice a week is needed. Babies can relieve entanglement and twisting. Those that cannot are vulnerable to problems that can be detected by fetal behavior monitoring and maternal awareness of the problem.

By twenty-six to twenty-eight weeks, the baby establishes its behavior patterns. A common pattern is for the baby to move at bedtime once the mother becomes supine. This event causes maternal blood flow shifts that the baby detects. It responds with reflex movement to reestablish its blood flow. This intrauterine reflex is a reliable sign of a healthy baby. If the baby moves a lot (hyperactivity) or moves less than normal, the mom should be evaluated on labor and delivery at that time. Taking these steps will be the best chance of achieving a live birth where UCA exists.

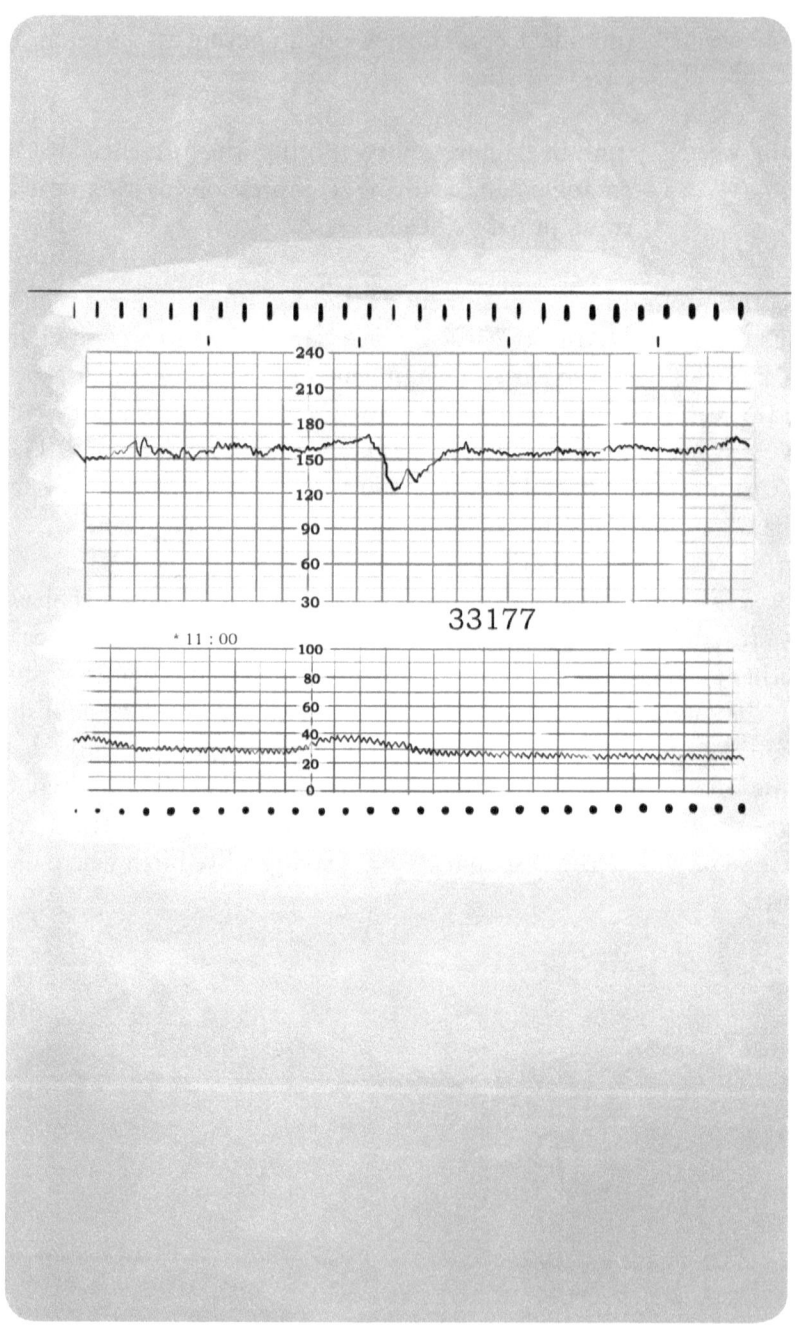

Non-stress test W sign decel

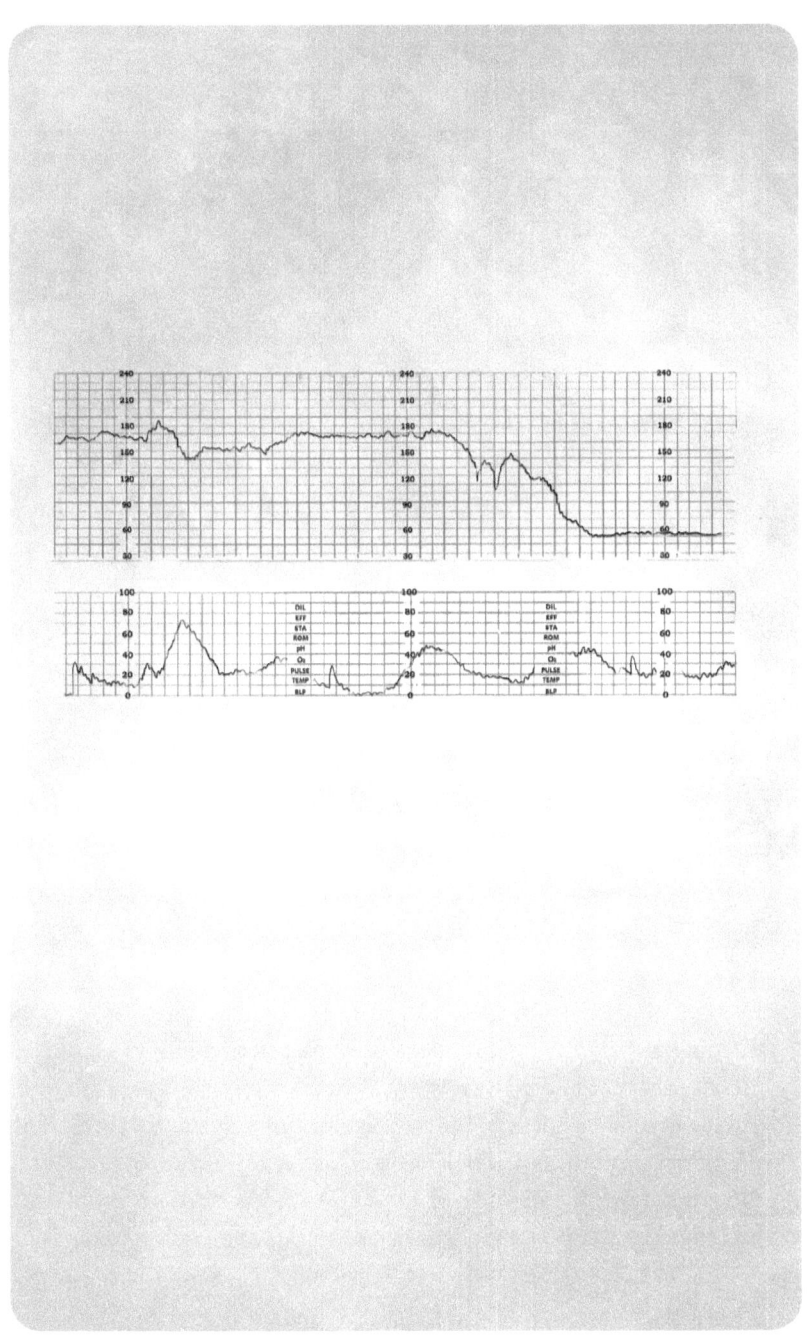

Fetal heart rate decline after W sign due to umbilical cord accident

Dr. J. Collins is from New Orleans, Louisiana, and trained with Tulane Medical Center. He specializes in obstetrics and gynecology. He recently completed a master's degree in clinical research from Tulane Medical Center. He is the principal investigator for the PUCP (Perinatal Umbilical Cord Project). The study reviewed over one thousand no-risk pregnancies for UCA and is peer reviewed and published by the Royal College of Obstetrics and Gynecology.

RECOMMENDED READING

Amiel-Tison, Claudine and Ann Stewart, eds. *The Newborn Infant: One Brain for Life*. Published by the National Institute of Health and Medical Research. Paris, France. 1994.

"Ann Jillian's Miracle Baby—Delivery Room Drama" (with a triple nuchal cord discovered at C-section). *National Enquirer* (February 25, 1992).

Arvy, L. and G. Pillepi, eds. 1976. "Le Cordon Ombilical (Fonis Umbilicalis)." Ostermundigen, Switzerland.

Atlas, Jan, ed. 2010. *They Were Still Born*. (Amazon.com).

Benirschke, Kurt and Peter Kaufman. 1990. *Pathology of the Human Placenta*. 2nd ed. New York, New York: Springer-Verlag.

Birnholz, Jason C. 1990. "Ecologic Physiology of the Fetus, Ultrasonography of Supply-Line Deprivations Syndromes." Radiologic Clinics of North America 28 (1): 179.

Brier, B. The murder of Tutankhamon, Berkeley Books NY, 1999, 116-117

Bukowski, R. et al. 2011. "Causes of Death Among Stillbirths." *Journal of the American Medical Association* 306 (22): 2459-2468. doi:10.1001/jama.2011.1823.

Cabaniss, Miki L., ed. 1993. *Fetal Monitoring Interpretation*. Philadelphia, Pennsylvania: J. B. Lippincott Co.

Clark, SL. et. al. 2013 Intrapartum Management of Category II heart rate tracings: Towards Standardization of Care. American Journal of Obstetrics and Gynecology 209.

Clapp, James F., III et. al. 1988. "Brain Damage After Intermittent Partial Cord Occlusion in the Chronically Instrumented Fetal Lamb." *American Journal of Obstetrics and Gynecology* 159: 504.

Collins, J. H. 2002. "Umbilical Cord Accidents: Human Studies." *Semin Perinatol* 26 (1): 79-82.

Collins, J. H. 2012. BMC Pregnancy and Childbirth 12 (Suppl 1): A7. http://www.biomedcentral.com/1471-2393/12/S1/A7.

Collins, J. H. and C. L. Collins. Edited by J. Kingdom, E. Jauniaux, and S. O'Brien. "The Human Umbilical Cord." In *The Placenta: Basic Science and Clinical Practice* 2000: 319-329. Ch 26. London: RCOG Press.

Collins, J.H., C. L. Collins, and C. C. Collins. 2010. "Umbilical Cord Accidents." http://www.preginst.com/UmbilicalCordAccidents2.pdf.

Corkill, T. F. 1961. "The Infant's Vulnerable Life-Line." *Australian New Zealand Journal of Obstetrics and Gynecology* 1: 154.

De Hann, Harmen H. et. al. 1997. "Brief Repeated Umbilical Cord Occlusions Cause Sustained Cytotoxic Cerebral Edema and Focal Infarcts in Near-Term Fetal Lambs." *Pediatric Research* 41: 96.

Harman, Christopher R., ed. 1995. *Invasive Fetal Testing and Treatment*. Winnipeg, Canada: Blackwell Scientific Publications. ISBN 0-86542-208-7.

Heifetz, S.A. Edited by S. H. Lewis and E. Perrin. "Pathology of the Umbilical Cord." In *Pathology of the Placenta*. 2nd ed. 1999: 1007-136. New York, New York: Churchill Livingstone.

Hon, Edward. 1969. "Watching the Unborn Inside the Womb: High Risk Mothers and the Graph that Raises Their Babies' Chances." *Life Magazine* (July 25) 63-66.

Kevin Kanty—"Death Before Life, An Account of Stillbirth due to Umbilical Cord Torsion." *Vogue* (May 1995) 93-96.

Kohner, Nancy and Alix Henley. 1995. *When a Baby Dies: The Experience of Late Miscarriage, Stillbirth, and Neonatal Death*. San Francisco, California: Harper Collins Publishers. ISBN 004-440-934-6.

Lee, ST, HON EH. Fetal hemodynamic response to umbilical cord compression. Obstet Gynecol 1963, 22: 553-562.

Mann, Leon. 1986. "Pregnancy Events and Brain Damage." *American Journal of Obstetrics and Gynecology* 155: 6.

Murata, Yuji et. al. 1994. "Variable Fetal Heart Rate Decelerations and Electrocortical Activities." *American Journal of Obstetrics and Gynecology* 170: 689.

Naeye, Richard L. 1992. *Disorders of the Placenta, Fetus, and Neonate: Diagnosis and Clinical Significance*. St. Louis, Missouri: Mosby Year Book.

Nathanielsz, Peter W. 1992. *Life Before Birth and a Time to be Born*. Ithaca, New York: Promethean Press.

Nelson, Karin B. and Jonas H. Ellenberg. *Antecedents of Cerebral Palsy*. National Institute of Neurological and Communicative Disorders and Stroke.

Nijhuis, J. G., ed. 1992. *Fetal Behaviour: Developmental and Perinatal Aspects*. Oxford, England: Oxford University Press.

Nilsson, Lennart. Text by Lars Hamberger. 1993. *A Child is Born*. New York: Bantam Doubleday Dell Publishing Group Inc. ISBN 0-440-50691-3.

Pfaffin, ed. 1994. *Annals of the New York Academy of Sciences* 736.

Reynolds, Samuel R. 1952. "The Umbilical Cord." *Scientific American* 187 (July): 70.

Ryan, W. D. et. al. "Placental Histologic Criteria for Diagnosis of Cord Accident: Sensitivity and Specificity." *Pediatric and Developmental Pathology* 2012 (15): 275-80. Department of Pathology University of San Diego, California.

Sadovsky, E. et. al. "Decreased Fetal Movements Associated with Umbilical Cord Complications." Israel. JMed Sci 1977 Mar; 13 (3): 295-8 ISR.

Simpson, Joe Leigh and Sherman Elias, eds. 1994. *Fetal Cells in Maternal Blood: Prospects for Noninvasive Prenatal Diagnosis*. New York, New York: New York Academy of Sciences.

Smotherman, William P. and Scott R. Robinson. 1988. *Behavior of the Fetus*. Caldwell, New Jersey: Telford Press.

Strong, Tom H. 1993. "Non-Coiled Umbilical Cord Vessels: A New Marker for the Fetus at Risk." *Obstetrics and Gynecology* 81: 409.

"Today's Latest Coo—Deborah Norville's Delivery" (which includes an umbilical cord knot). *People* (March 25, 1991) 67-73.

Torpin, Richard. 1974. *Reproduction in Man and His Ancestors for 700 Million Years*. McGowen Printing Company.

Townsend, Jessica, ed. 1992. *Strengthening Research in Academic Ob/Gyn Departments*. Washington, DC: National Academy Press.

Wilson, B. 2008. "Sonography of the Placenta and Umbilical Cord." *Radiologic Technology* 79 (4): 333-345S.

Recommended Professional Reading

Professional Reading

References:

1. Montague, C.F., *Short Umbilical Cord Complicating Elective Pitocin Induction.* California Medicine, 1960. 93(1): p. 38-39.

2. Tantbirojn, P., et al., *Gross abnormalities of the umbilical cord: Related placental histology and clinical significance.* Placenta, 2009.

3. Parast, M.M., C.P. Crum, and T.K. Boyd, *Placental histologic criteria for umbilical blood flow restriction in unexplained stillbirth.* Hum Pathol, 2008. 39(6): p. 948-53.

4. Niswander, K., Gordon M., edts, *The Collaborative Perinatal Study of the National Institute of Neurological Diseases and Stroke,* in *The Women and Their Pregnancies W B Saunders.* 1972: Philadelphia PA.

5. *Physician Insurers Association of America. Neurologic Impairment in newborns; A Malpractice Claim Study.* PIAA Publ; 1998; Rockville, MD

6. Schindler, N.R., *Importance of the placenta and cord in the defense of neurologically impaired infant claims.* Arch Pathol Lab Med, 1991. 7: p. 685-687.

7. Naeye, R.L., *Disorders of the umbilical cord.* In in *Disorders of the Placenta, Fetus, and Neonate: Diagnosis and Clinical Significance.* 1992, Mosby Year Book St. Louis Inc; MO: 92-117.

8. Spellacy, W.N., Gravem BA, Fisch RO, *The umbilical cord complications of true knots, nuchal coils, and cords around the body.* Am J Obstet Gynecol, 1966. 94: p. 1136-1142.

9. Naeye, R.L., *Causes of Perinatal Mortality in the US Collaborative Perinatal Project.* JAMA, 1977. 238: p. 228-229.

10. Arvy, L. and G. Pilleri, *Le Cordon Ombilical, funis umbilicalis.* 1976 Ostermundigen: Bern, Switzerland.

11. Blackburn, W. and R.C. Nelson, *The Umbilical Cord.* Human Malformations and Related Anomalies, ed. R.E. Stevenson and J.G. hall. Vol. II. 1993. 1081-1141, N.Y., N.Y.: Oxford University Press.

12. Heifetz, S.A., *Pathology of the umbilical cord* Pathology of the Placenta (ed 2), ed. S.H. Lewis and E. Perrin. 1999. 1007-136, N.Y., N.Y.: Churchill Livingstone.

13. Benirschke, K. and P. Kaufmann, *Pathology of the Human Placenta, (ed 4).* 2000, N.Y., N.Y.: Springer-Verlag.

14. Blackburn, W., ed. *Umbilical Cord.* second ed. Human Malformations and Related Anomalies, ed. J.G.H. Roger E Stevenson 2006, Oxford University Press: New York. 1413-1472.

15. Keeling JW, K.T.e., ed. *Fetal and Neonatal Pathology.* 4th ed. 2007, Springer-Verlag: London. 54-76.

16. Towers, C.V., C.E. Juratsch, and T.J. Garite, *The fetal heart monitor tracing in pregnancies complicated by a spontaneous umbilical cord hematoma.* J Perinatol, 2009. 29(7): p. 517-20.

17. Bord, A., S. Yagel, and D.V. Valsky, *Overburdened and undernourished.* Am J Obstet Gynecol, 2007. 197(3): p. 324 e1-2.

18. Itakura, A., et al., *Intrauterine growth retardation and fetal distress associated with the excessively long (160*

cm) umbilical cord. Arch Gynecol Obstet, 1994. 255(2): p. 99-100.

19. Sherer, D.M., et al., *Power Doppler and 3-dimensional sonographic diagnosis of multiple separate true knots of the umbilical cord.* J Ultrasound Med, 2005. 24(9): p. 1321-3.

20. Smith, S., *A Case of Homicidal Strangulation of a Foetus by the Umbilical Cord.* The Lancet, 1927. 210(5432): p. 755-756.

21. Cotzias, C.S., Paterson-Brown S, Fisk NM, *Prospective risk of unexplained stillbirth in singleton pregnancies at term: population based analysis.* BMJ, 1999. 319: p. 287-288.

22. *CESDI 6th Annual Report. Maternal and Child Health Research Consortium.* 1997: London, England.

23. Froen, J.F., Arnestad M, Frey K, Vege A, Saugstad OD, Stray-Pedersen B, *Risk factors for the sudden intrauterine unexplained death: Epidemiologic characteristics of singleton cases in Oslo, Norway, 1986-1995.* Am J Obstet Gynecol, 2001. 184: p. 694-702.

24. Weeks, J.W., Asrat T, Morgan MA, Nageotte M, Thomas SJ, Freeman RK, *Antepartum surveillance for a history of stillbirth: When to begin.* Am J Obstet Gynecol, 1995. 172: p. 486-492.

25. Gabor, J., et al., *Harmadik Trimestererbeli intrauterin magzati elhlasok.* Orvosi Hetilap, 1999. 140: p. 2399-2402.

26. Kunzel, W., *Intrauterine Fetal Death during Pregnancy: Limitations of Fetal Surveillance.* J Obstet Gynecol, 1998. 24: p. 453-60.

27. Konchak, P.S., Billman BD, Walczak JR, *Stillbirth: Maternal and fetal evaluation.* JAOA, 1989. 89: p. 1150-57.

28. Dombrowski, M.P., et al., *Ultrasound findings in gestations destined for unanticipated fetal demise.* Ultrasound Obstet Gynecol, 1991. 1(4): p. 269-71.

29. Archibong, E.I., A.A. Sobande, and A.A. Asindi, *Antenatal intrauterine fetal death: a prospective study in a tertiary hospital in south-western Saudi Arabia.* J Obstet Gynaecol, 2003. 23(2): p. 170-3.

30. Collins, J.H., Collins CL, *The Human Umbilical Cord.* The Placenta: Basic Science and Clinical Practice, ed. J. Kingdom, E. Jauniaux, and S. O'Brien. 2000. Ch 26 pp 319-329, London: RCOG Press.

31. Domenighetti, C., Paccaund F, *The Night-a dangerous time to be born?* Br J Obstet Gynaecol, 1986. 93: p. 1262-1267.

32. Seron-Ferre, M., Riffo R, Valenzuela GJ, Germain AM, *Twenty-four-hour pattern of cortisol in the human fetus at term.* Am J Obstet Gynecol, 2001. 184: p. 1278-1283.

33. Smotherman, W.P. and S.R. Robinson, eds. *Behavior of the Fetus.* 1988, The Telford Press: Caldwell, NJ.

34. Nathanielsz, P.W., *Life Before Birth and A Time to Be Born.* 1992, Ithaca, NY: Promethean Press.

35. Lunshof, M.S., *Circadian rhythms in the normal and growth-retarded fetus and infant.* 2000, University of Amsterdam; Amsterdam, The Netherlands.

36. Stewart, J.H., J. Andrews, and P.H. Cartlidge, *Numbers of deaths related to intrapartum asphyxia and timing of birth in all Wales perinatal survey, 1993-5.* BMJ, 1998. 316(7132): p. 657-60.

37. Gould, J.B., C. Qin, and G. Chavez, *Time of birth and the risk of neonatal death.* Obstet Gynecol, 2005. 106(2): p. 352-8.

38. Minors, D.S. and J.M. Waterhouse, *Circadian rhythms in general.* Occup Med, 1990. 5(2): p. 165-82.

39. Tan, K.C., N.K. Ho, and B.L. Tay, *Stillbirths--ten years experience at Toa Payoh Hospital.* Singapore Med J, 1989. 30(2): p. 151-4.

40. Incerpi, M.H., Miller DA, Samadi R, Settlage RH, Goodwin TM, *Stillbirth evaluation: what tests are needed?* Am J Obstet Gynecol, 1998. 178: p. 1121-25.

41. Baergen, R.N., *Cord abnormalities, structural lesions, and cord "accidents".* Semin Diagn Pathol, 2007. 24(1): p. 23-32.

42. Alessandri, L.M., Stanley FJ, Garner JB, Newnham J, Walters BNJ, *A case-control study of unexplained antepartum stillbirth.* Br J Obstet and Gynaecol, 1992. 99: p. 711-18.

43. Oron, T., Sheiner E, Shoham-Vardi I, Mazor M, Katz M, Hallak M, *Risk factors for antepartum fetal death.* J Reprod Med, 2001. 46: p. 825-30.

44. Adams, M., *Validity of Birth Certificate Data for the Outcome of the Previous Pregnancy Georgia, 1980-1995.* American Journal of Epidemiology, 2001. 154(10): p. 883-888.

45. Larciprete, G., et al., *Absent end diastolic flow in umbilical artery and umbilical cord thrombosis at term of pregnancy.* Med Sci Monit, 2003. 9(5): p. CS29-33.

46. Bohm, W. and C. Zenk, *[Significance of umbilical cord anomalies within the frame of perinatal mortality].* Zentralbl Gynakol, 1976. 98(8): p. 475-80.

47. Ogunyemi, D., Jackson U, Buyske S, Risk A, *Clinical and pathologic correlations of stillbirth in a single institution.* Acta Obstet Gynecol Scand, 1998. 77: p. 722-728.

48. Huang, D.Y., *Determinants of Unexplained Antepartum Fetal Deaths.* Am J Obstet Gynecol, 2000. 95(2): p. 215-21.

49. Clausen, I., *Umbilical cord anomalies and antenatal fetal deaths.* Obstet Gynecol Surv, 1989. 44(12): p. 841-5.

50. Corkill, T.F., *The infant's vulnerable life-line.* Aust N Z J Obstet Gynecol, 1961. 1: p. 154-60.

51. Wessel, J., Gerhold W, Unger M, Lichteneger W, Vogel M, *Umbilical cord complications as a cause of intrauterine death.* Z Geburtshilfe Perinatol 1992. 196: p. 173-76.

52. Ghosh, A., Woo JSK, MacHenry C, Wan CW, O'Hoy KM, MA HK, *Fetal loss from umbilical cord abnormalities-a difficult case for prevention* Europ J Obstet Gynec Reprod Biol, 1984. 18: p. 183-98.

53. Mesleh, R.A., et al., *Changing trends in perinatal deaths at the Armed Forces Hospital, Riyadh, Saudi Arabia.* J Obstet Gynaecol, 2001. 21(1): p. 49-55.

54. Jouan, H., et al., *[Pathology of the umbilical cord].* Arch Anat Cytol Pathol, 1983. 31(3): p. 148-53.

55. Heifetz, S.A., *The umbilical cord: obstetrically important lesions.* Clin Obstet Gynecol, 1996. 39(3): p. 571-87.

56. Aspillaga, C., et al., *[Anomalies of the umbilical cord and its association with fetal malformations].* Rev Chil Obstet Ginecol, 1991. 56(1): p. 27-34.

57. Mortensen, E. and M.S. Kearney, *Meconium aspiration in the mid trimester fetus: an autopsy study.* Pediatr Dev Pathol, 2009: p. 1.

58. Korteweg, F.J., et al., *Diverse placental pathologies as the main causes of fetal death.* Obstet Gynecol, 2009. 114(4): p. 809-17.

59. Fretts, R., *Management of Stillbirth.* ACOG Practice Bulletin, 2009. 102(March).

60. Kirkup, B., Welch G, *"Normal but dead": perinatal mortality in non-malformed babies of birthweight 2.5 kg and over in the Northern Region in 1983.* Br J Obstet Gynaecol, 1990. 97: p. 381-392.

61. Lee, K.S., Khoshnood B, Chen L, Wall SN, Cromie WJ, Mittendorf RL, *Infant Mortality From Congenital Malformations in the United States, 1970-1997.* Obstet Gynecol, 2001. 98: p. 620-627.

62. Holly B. Ford, D.J.S., *Recurrent Pregnancy Loss: Etiology, Diagnosis, and Therapy.* Reviews in Obstetrics & Gynecology, 2009. 2(2): p. 76-83.

63. Baena, N., et al., *Fetal and placenta chromosome constitution in 237 pregnancy losses.* Ann Genet, 2001. 44(2): p. 83-8.

64. McClure, E.M. and R.L. Goldenberg, *Infection and stillbirth.* Semin Fetal Neonatal Med, 2009. 14(4): p. 182-9.

65. Wiedersberg, E., G. Wittstock, and H. Wiedersberg, *Pathology of the umbilical cord in relation to gestational age: findings in 4,267 fetal and neonatal autopsies.* Verh Dtsch Ges Pathol, 2001. 85: p. 175-92.

66. Javert, C.T., Barton B, *Congenital and acquired lesions of the umbilical cord and spontaneous abortion.* Am J Obstet Gynecol, 1952. 63: p. 1065-1073.

67. Frkovic, A., Randic L, Krstuljia M, *Fetal Death during 20th to 36th week of pregnancy.* Jugosi Ginekol Perinatol, 1990. 30: p. 23-26.

68. Wiedersberg, E., G. Wittstock, and H. Wiedersberg, *Pathologie der Nabelschnur in Abhangigkeit vom Gestationsalter. Befunde bei 4267 fetalen und neonatalen Autopsien.* Verh Dtsch Ges Pathol, 2001. 85: p. 185-192.

69. Collins, J.H., Collins CL, *What is Shoulder Dystocia?* J Reprod Med, 2001. 46: p. 148-150.

70. Sabai, B.M., ed. *Hypertensive Disorders in Women.* 2001: W B Saunders, Philadelphia, PA.

71. Gallot, D., H. Laurichesse, and D. Lemery, *Selective feticide in monochorionic twin pregnancies by ultrasound-guided umbilical cord occlusion.* Ultrasound Obstet Gynecol, 2003. 22(5): p. 484-8.

72. Robyr, R., M. Yamamoto, and Y. Ville, *Selective feticide in complicated monochorionic twin pregnancies using ultrasound-guided bipolar cord coagulation.* BJOG, 2005. 112(10): p. 1344-8.

73. Rossi, A.C. and V. D'Addario, *Umbilical cord occlusion for selective feticide in complicated monochorionic twins: a systematic review of literature.* Am J Obstet Gynecol, 2009. 200(2): p. 123-9.

74. Bako, B., C. Chama, and B.M. Audu, *Emergency obstetrics care in a Nigerian tertiary hospital: a 20 year review of umblical cord prolapse.* Niger J Clin Pract, 2009. 12(3): p. 232-6.

75. Khan, R.S., T. Naru, and F. Nizami, *Umbilical cord prolapse--a review of diagnosis to delivery interval on perinatal and maternal outcome.* J Pak Med Assoc, 2007. 57(10): p. 487-91.

76. Dufour, P., et al., *[Cord prolapse. Review of the literature. A series of 50 cases].* J Gynecol Obstet Biol Reprod (Paris), 1996. 25(8): p. 841-5.

77. Dilbaz, B., et al., *Risk factors and perinatal outcomes associated with umbilical cord prolapse.* Arch Gynecol Obstet, 2006. 274(2): p. 104-7.

78. Kahana, B., et al., *Umbilical cord prolapse and perinatal outcomes.* Int J Gynaecol Obstet, 2004. 84(2): p. 127-32.

79. Traore, Y., et al., *[Frequency of cord prolapse: etiological factors and fetal prognosis in 47 cases in a health center].* Mali Med, 2006. 21(1): p. 25-9.

80. Middeldorp, J.M., et al., *Selective feticide in monoamniotic twin pregnancies by umbilical cord occlusion and transection.* Fetal Diagn Ther, 2008. 23(2): p. 121-5.

81. Miura, N. and S. Suzuki, *Fetal asphyxia due to cord entanglement in a monochorionic diamniotic twin pregnancy complicated by 2nd-trimester single intrauterine demise.* Fetal Diagn Ther, 2008. 23(1): p. 69-71.

82. Dickinson, J.E., *Monoamniotic twin pregnancy: a review of contemporary practice.* Aust N Z J Obstet Gynaecol, 2005. 45(6): p. 474-8.

83. Leeners, B., et al., *Reversible absent/reversed end-diastolic flow in the umbilical artery, and reversible brain-sparing effect in a case with umbilical cord entanglement.* Prenat Diagn, 2005. 25(6): p. 516-8.

84. Redline, R.W., *Clinical and pathological umbilical cord abnormalities in fetal thrombotic vasculopathy.* Hum Pathol, 2004. 35(12): p. 1494-8.

85. de Laat, M.W., et al., *Hypercoiling of the umbilical cord and placental maturation defect: associated pathology?* Pediatr Dev Pathol, 2007. 10(4): p. 293-9.

86. Christoforidis, N., E. Gouk, and M. Roberts, *Cardiotocography in umbilical cord entanglement.* J Obstet Gynaecol, 1998. 18(6): p. 590-1.

87. Blackburn, W., et al., *An evaluation and classification of the lesions attending abnormal surface encounters with the fetal habitat.* Proc Greenwood Genet Center, 1997. 6: p. 81-89.

88. Juhasz, G., et al., *[Intrauterine fetal death in the third trimester].* Orv Hetil, 1999. 140(43): p. 2399-402.

89. Carey, J.C. and W.F. Rayburn, *Nuchal cord encirclements and risk of stillbirth.* Int J Gynaecol Obstet, 2000. 69(2): p. 173-4.

90. Holt, J., et al., *Perinatal deaths in a Norwegian county 1986-96 classified by the Nordic-Baltic perinatal classification: geographical contrasts as a basis for quality assessment.* Acta Obstet Gynecol Scand, 2000. 79(2): p. 107-12.

91. Serinius, F., Winbo I, Dahlquist G, Kallen B, *Cause-specific stillbirth and neonatal death in Sweden: a catchment area-based analysis.* Acta Paediatr, 2001. 90: p. 1054-1061.

92. Serinius, F., Winbo I, Dahlquist G, Kallen B, *Regional differences in stillbirth and neonatal death rate in Sweden with a cause-of-death specific analysis.* Acta Paediatr, 2001. 90: p. 1062-1067.

93. Jouan H, e.a., *The Pathology of the Umbilical Cord.* Sem. Hop. Paris 1983. 59(43): p. 3003-3008.

94. Aldo J, G.M., *Significacion Clinica de la Patologia del Cordon Umbilical.* Revista de Obstetrica y Ginecologia de Venezuela, 1967. 27(3): p. 459-81.

95. Yeong, C.T., et al., *Optimising management of stillbirths in modern Singapore.* Singapore Med J, 1997. 38(8): p. 317-20.

96. Gai, M.Y., *[Intrauterine deaths: a clinical and pathologic analysis].* Zhonghua Fu Chan Ke Za Zhi, 1990. 25(5): p. 282-4, 316.

97. Abbott, F.F., *An Anomaly of the Umbilical Cord.* California and Western Medicine, 1931. XXXV (2): p. 126-127.

98. Avagliano, L., et al., *Thrombosis of the umbilical vessels revisited. An observational study of 317 consecutive autopsies at a single institution.* Hum Pathol, 2010.

99. Hatch, M.C., Schoeneck FJ, *Perinatal Mortality Caused by Cord Complications, Pathology and Management.* New York State Journal of Medicine, 1965. Feb: p. 433-436.

100. Lillien, A., *Term Intrapartum Fetal Death.* Am J Obstet Gynecol, 1970. 107: p. 595-603.

101. Sebire, N.J. and W. Sepulveda, *Correlation of placental pathology with prenatal ultrasound findings.* J Clin Pathol, 2008. 61(12): p. 1276-84.

102. Kidron, D., J. Bernheim, and R. Aviram, *Placental findings contributing to fetal death, a study of 120 stillbirths between 23 and 40 weeks gestation.* Placenta, 2009. 30(8): p. 700-4.

103. Amir, H., *A Piece of the Puzzle of IUFD: Pathological Findings in Placentas From Term and Preterm IUFD*

Pregnancies. American Journal of Obstetrics & Gynecology, 2008. 119-Suppl(Abst 374): p. S113.

104. Randall, G.C.B., *Form and development of the umbilical cord in pigs and their association with the delivery of viable pigs.* Am J Vet Res, 1989. 50: p. 1512-1515.

105. Whitwell, K.E., *Morphology and Pathology of the Equine Umbilical Cord.* J Reprod Fert, Suppl, 1975. 23: p. 599-603.

106. Brady, A.G., *Knotted umbilical cord as a cause of death in a Cercopithhecus aethiops fetus.* Lab Anim Sci, 1983. 1983(33): p. 375-376.

107. Pospichil, A., Lieb A, Corboz L, *Causes of prenatal foal loss in Switzerland.* Schweiz Arch Tierheilkd, 1992. 134: p. 401-9.

108. Giles, R.C., Donahue JM, Hong CB, Tuttle PA, Petrites-Murphy MB, Poonacha KB, et al, *Causes of abortion, stillbirth, and perinatal death in horses: 3,527 cases (1986-1991).* J Am Vet Assoc, 1993. 15: p. 1170-75.

109. Wilsher, S., J. Ousey, and W.R. Allen, *Abnormal umbilical cord attachment sites in the mare: a review illustrated by three case reports.* Equine Vet J, 2009. 41(9): p. 930-9.

110. Wang, G., Bove KE, Stank J, *Pathologic Evidence of prolonged umbilical cord encirclement as a cause of fetal death.* Am J Perinatol, 1998. 15: p. 585-588.

111. Lin, A.E., Genest DR, Brown DL, *Circumferential abdominal skin defect possibly due to umbilical cord encirclement.* Teratology, 1999. 60: p. 258-9.

112. Minakami, H., Akahori A, Sakurai S, Yamauchi A, Sato I, *Umbilical vein thrombosis as a possible cause of perinatal*

morbidity or mortality: report of two cases. J Obstet Gynaecol Res, 2001. 27: p. 97-101.

113. Brewster, J.A., Quenby SM, Alfirevic Z, *Intra-uterine death due to umbilical cord thrombosis secondary to antiphospholipid syndrome.* Lupus, 1999. 8(558-559).

114. Tuggle, A.Q., Cook WA, *Laceration of a placental vein: An injury possibly inflicted by the fetus.* Am J Obstet Gynecol, 1978. 131: p. 220-221.

115. Malin, G.L., R.K. Morris, and K.S. Khan, *Strength of association between umbilical cord pH and perinatal and long term outcomes: systematic review and meta-analysis.* BMJ, 2010. 340: p. c1471.

116. Romero, R., Chervenak FA, Coustan D, Berkowitz RL, Hobbins JC, *Antenatal sonographic diagnosis of umbilical cord laceration.* Am J Obstet Gynecol, 1982. 143: p. 719-20.

117. Tischendorf, D., *Umbilical cord complications as the cause for intrauterine death.* Zentralbl Gynakol, 1977. 99: p. 234-239.

118. Yamauchi, A., et al., *Causes of stillbirth: an analysis of 77 cases.* J Obstet Gynaecol Res, 1999. 25(6): p. 419-24.

119. Franciosi, R.A., *Placental pathology casebook. Chorangiosis of the placenta increases the probability of perinatal mortality.* J Perinatol, 1999. 19(5): p. 393-4.

120. Eizenberg, D., *Antenatal true umbilical cord knot leading to fetal demise.* Aust N Z J Obstet Gynaecol, 1998. 38(1): p. 100-1.

121. Corridan, M., E.D. Kendall, and J.D. Begg, *Cord entanglement causing premature placental separation and*

amniotic fluid embolism. Case report. Br J Obstet Gynaecol, 1980. 87(11): p. 935-40.

122. Capponi, A., et al., *The effects of fetal blood sampling and placental puncture on umbilical artery and fetal arterial vessels blood flow velocity waveforms.* Am J Perinatol, 1996. 13(3): p. 185-90.

123. Teixeira, J.M., V. Glover, and N.M. Fisk, *Acute cerebral redistribution in response to invasive procedures in the human fetus.* Am J Obstet Gynecol, 1999. 181(4): p. 1018-25.

124. Hertogs, K., et al., *The safety of fetoscopy: (I). Effect of umbilical vessel puncture on the fetal heart rate and cord histology.* Prenat Diagn, 1983. 3(2): p. 91-6.

125. Patten, R.M., et al., *Twin embolization syndrome: prenatal sonographic detection and significance.* Radiology, 1989. 173(3): p. 685-9.

126. Okamura, K., et al., *Funipuncture for evaluation of hematologic and coagulation indices in the surviving twin following co-twin's death.* Obstet Gynecol, 1994. 83(6): p. 975-8.

127. Cave, D.G., Swingler GR, Skew PG, *Hypoxic stillbirth due to entangled intrauterine catheter.* BMJ, 1979. 27: p. 233.

128. Trudinger, B.J., Pryse-Davies J, *Fetal Hazards of the Intrauterine Pressure Catheter: Five Case Reports.* Br J Obstet and Gynaecol, 1978. 85: p. 567-572.

129. Gupta, I., V.F. Hillier, and J.M. Edwards, *Multiple vascular profiles in the umbilical cord; an indication of maternal smoking habits and intrauterine distress.* Placenta, 1993. 14(1): p. 117-23.

130. Candussi, G., G. Carlomagno, and R. Bussani, *[Analysis of a case of umbilical cord abnormalities associated with fetal death]*. Minerva Ginecol, 1987. 39(6): p. 413-5.

131. Buchsbaum, J.H., *Accidental injury complicating pregnancy*. Am J Obstet Gynecol, 1968. 102: p. 752.

132. Goodlin, R.C. and W.H. Clewell, *Sudden fetal death following diagnostic amniocentesis*. Am J Obstet Gynecol, 1974. 118(2): p. 285.

133. Emura, T., et al., *Omphalocele associated with a large multilobular umbilical cord pseudocyst*. Pediatr Surg Int, 2004. 20(8): p. 636-9.

134. Wigglesworth, J.S., *Classification of perinatal deaths*. Soz Praventivmed, 1994. 39(1): p. 11-4.

135. Weill, R. and E. Girard, *[Multiple tightened coils with fetal death in successive pregnancies.]*. Bull Fed Soc Gynecol Obstet Lang Fr, 1957. 9(2): p. 192-3.

136. Vermelin, M.H., *Multiples serres avec mort foetale a repetition*. Societe D'Obstetrique et Gynecologie de Nancy, 1956(April): p. 192-4.

137. Getahun, D., et al., *The association between stillbirth in the first pregnancy and subsequent adverse perinatal outcomes*. Am J Obstet Gynecol, 2009. 201(4): p. 378 e1-6.

138. Lykke, J.A., M.J. Paidas, and J. Langhoff-Roos, *Recurring complications in second pregnancy*. Obstet Gynecol, 2009. 113(6): p. 1217-24.

139. Ananth, C.V., et al., *Recurrence of fetal growth restriction in singleton and twin gestations*. J Matern Fetal Neonatal Med, 2009: p. 1-8.

140. Kwok, W., *Recurrent Multiple Chorangiomas and Intrauterine Death.* Pathology, 1988. 20: p. 77-78.

141. Semchyshyn, S., *True knot of the umbilical cord in two consecutive pregnancies.* CMA Journal, 1973. 109: p. 269.

142. Bakotic, B.W., et al., *Recurrent umbilical cord torsion leading to fetal death in 3 subsequent pregnancies: a case report and review of the literature.* Arch Pathol Lab Med, 2000. 124(9): p. 1352-5.

143. Baergen, R.N., et al., *Morbidity, mortality, and placental pathology in excessively long umbilical cords: retrospective study.* Pediatr Dev Pathol, 2001. 4(2): p. 144-53.

144. Weeks, J.W., *Antepartum testing for women with previous stillbirth.* Semin Perinatol, 2008. 32(4): p. 301-6.

145. Collins, J.H., et al., *Nuchal cords: timing of antenatal diagnosis and duration.* Am J Obstet Gynecol, 1995. 173(3 Pt 1): p. 768.

146. Larson, J.D., W.F. Rayburn, and V.L. Harlan, *Nuchal cord entanglement and gestational age.* Am J Perinatol, 1997. 14(9): p. 555-57.

147. Nijhuis, J.G., ed. *Fetal Behavior Developmental and Perinatal Aspects.* 1992, Oxford University Press: Oxford, England.

148. Collins, J.H., *Home Fetal Monitoring After Previous Stillbirth Due to Umbilical Cord Accident*, in *Society for Fetal Physiology*. 2007. p. 1.

149. Heinonen, S. and P. Kirkinen, *Pregnancy outcomes after previous stillbirth resulting from causes other than maternal conditions and fetal abnormalities.* Birth, 2000. 27: p. 3-37.

150. Samueloff, A., et al., *Recurrent stillbirth. Significance and characteristics.* J Reprod Med, 1993. 38(11): p. 883-6.

151. Whitley, E., *Graphical trees: the simultaneous display of risk of fetal death by pregnancy history and maternal age.* Paediatr Perinat Epidemiol, 1999. 13(3): p. 342-51.

152. Reddy, U.M., *Prediction and prevention of recurrent stillbirth.* Obstet Gynecol, 2007. 110(5): p. 1151-64.

153. Beurton D. H J, Q.F., Deugnier Y, Kerisit J, *The pathology of the umbilical cord.* Sem. Hop. Paris, 1983. 59(43): p. 3003-3008.

154. Giugni, A.J., *[Clinical meaning of the umbilical cord pathology].* Rev Obstet Ginecol Venez, 1967. 27(3): p. 459-81.

155. Blyumkin, V.N., *The Functional Significance of innervation of the human umbilical cord.* Bulletin of Experimental Biology and Medicine, 1957. 43(2): p. 223-226.

156. Ellison, J.P., *The nerves of the umbilical cord in man and the rat.* Am J Anat, 1971. 132(1): p. 53-60.

157. Marzioni, D., et al., *Restricted innervation of uterus and placenta during pregnancy: evidence for a role of the repelling signal Semaphorin 3A.* Dev Dyn, 2004. 231(4): p. 839-48.

158. Matsubara, S. and T. Tamada, *Presence of nerve fibers in the human umbilical cord--an electron microscopical histochemical proof.* Nippon Sanka Fujinka Gakkai Zasshi, 1988. 40(11): p. 1775-6.

159. Fox, H. and H.N. Jacobson, *Innervation of the human umbilical cord and umbilical vessels.* Am J Obstet Gynecol, 1969. 103(3): p. 384-9.

160. Nanaev, A.K., et al., *Stromal differentiation and architecture of the human umbilical cord.* Placenta, 1997. 18(1): p. 53-64.

161. Benedetto, C., et al., *Production of prostacyclin, 6-keto-PGF1 alpha and thromboxane B2 by human umbilical vessels increases from the placenta towards the fetus.* Br J Obstet Gynaecol, 1987. 94(12): p. 1165-9.

162. Franc, S., et al., *Microfibrillar composition of umbilical cord matrix: characterization of fibrillin, collagen VI and intact collagen V.* Placenta, 1998. 19(1): p. 95-104.

163. Masuda, M., et al., *Element content of human umbilical artery and vein in umbilical cord.* Biol Trace Elem Res, 1999. 69(3): p. 235-40.

164. Oudesluys Murphy, H.M., *The Human Umbilical Cord and its Separation.* 1990, Pedia Boek: Oud-Beijerland.

165. Martin de Llano, J.J., et al., *Birth weight and characteristics of endothelial and smooth muscle cell cultures from human umbilical cord vessels.* J Transl Med, 2009. 7: p. 30.

166. Sinnathuray, *The Vasomotor Response of the Human Umbilical Cord Vessels to Changes in its External Thermal Environment.* The Australian and New Zealand Journal of Obstetrics and Gynaecology, 1968. 8(3): p. 140-145.

167. Ruchira, S., et al., *Gene expression patterns in human placenta.* PNAS, 2006. 103(14): p. 5478-5483.

168. Turner, A.J. and B.J. Trudinger, *A modification of the uterine artery restriction technique in the guinea pig fetus produces asymmetrical ultrasound growth.* Placenta, 2009. 30(3): p. 236-40.

169. Aagaard-Tillery, K., et al., *Sample bias among women with retained DNA samples for future genetic studies.* Obstet Gynecol, 2006. 108(5): p. 1115-20.

170. Hussain, N., et al., *Effects of prenatal tobacco exposure on gene expression profiling in umbilical cord tissue.* Pediatr Res, 2008. 64(2): p. 147-53.

171. Cohen, J.e.a., *Umbilical cord gene expression signals premature babies' lung disease risk.* Genome Biology, 2007. 8(10): p. R210.

172. Rockelein, G. and R. Schneider, *Die dreidimensionale Analyse der Media der Umbilikalarterien.* Z Geburtsh u Perinat, 1992. 196: p. 266-272.

173. Vizza, E., et al., *The collagen fibrils arrangement in the Wharton's jelly of full-term human umbilical cord.* Ital J Anat Embryol, 1995. 100 Suppl 1: p. 495-501.

174. Morris, J.F. and A.C. Hunt, *Breaking strength of the umbilical cord.* J Forensic Sci, 1966. 11(1): p. 43-9.

175. Spann, W. and H.M. Englert, *[Experimental studies on the laceration resistance of the umbilical cord].* Dtsch Z Gesamte Gerichtl Med, 1967. 59(2): p. 196-200.

176. Crichton, J.L., *Tensile strength of the umbilical cord.* Am J Obstet Gynecol, 1973. 115(1): p. 77-80.

177. Frye, S.R., et al., *cDNA microarray analysis of endothelial cells subjected to cyclic mechanical strain: importance of motion control.* Physiol Genomics, 2005. 21(1): p. 124-30.

178. Gervaso, F., et al. *Biomechanics of the human umbilical cord under compressive loads.* in *2003 Summer Bioengineering Conference, June 25-29.* 2003. Sonesta Beach Resort in Key Biscayne, FL.

179. Ghosh, K.G., S.N. Ghosh, and A.B. Gupta, *Tensile properties of human umbilical cord.* Indian J Med Res, 1984. 79: p. 538-41.

180. Itskovitz, J., et al., *Intrauterine rupture of the umbilical cord during delivery.* Eur J Obstet Gynecol Reprod Biol, 1980. 10(1): p. 35-40.

181. Warm, R., *[Cord traction?].* Z Arztl Fortbild (Jena), 1972. 66(8): p. 407-10.

182. Langer, H., *[The pull on the umbilical cord].* Dtsch Med Wochenschr, 1968. 93(6): p. 246 passim.

183. Ghezzi, F., et al., *First-trimester umbilical cord diameter: a novel marker of fetal aneuploidy.* Ultrasound Obstet Gynecol, 2002. 19(3): p. 235-9.

184. Li, W.C., et al., *Biomechanical properties of different segments of human umbilical cord vein and its value for clinical application.* J Biomed Mater Res B Appl Biomater, 2006. 76(1): p. 93-7.

185. Kouvalainen, K., et al., *[Weights of placenta, fetal membranes and umbilical cord].* Duodecim, 1971. 87(17): p. 1210-4.

186. Weissman, A., et al., *Sonographic measurements of the umbilical cord and vessels during normal pregnancies.* J Ultrasound Med, 1994. 13(1): p. 11-4.

187. Moinian, M., W.W. Meyer, and J. Lind, *Diameters of umbilical cord vessels and the weight of the cord in relation to clamping time.* Am J Obstet Gynecol, 1969. 105(4): p. 604-11.

188. Patel, D., et al., *Umbilical cord circumference at birth.* Am J Dis Child, 1989. 143(6): p. 638-9.

189. Pennati, G., *Biomechanical properties of the human umbilical cord.* Biorheology, 2001. 38(5-6): p. 355-66.

190. Axt-Fliedner, R., et al., *Umbilical cord diameter at 11-14 weeks of gestation: relationship to nuchal translucency, ductus venous blood flow and chromosomal defects.* Fetal Diagn Ther, 2006. 21(4): p. 390-5.

191. Ghezzi, F., et al., *First-trimester sonographic umbilical cord diameter and the growth of the human embryo.* Ultrasound Obstet Gynecol, 2001. 18(4): p. 348-51.

192. Goynumer, G., et al., *Umbilical cord thickness in the first and early second trimesters and perinatal outcome.* J Perinat Med, 2008. 36(6): p. 523-6.

193. Barbieri, C., et al., *Inter- and intra-observer variability in Sonographic measurements of the cross-sectional diameters and area of the umbilical cord and its vessels during pregnancy.* Reprod Health, 2008. 5: p. 5.

194. Goodlin, R.C., *Fetal dysmaturity, "lean cord," and fetal distress.* Am J Obstet Gynecol, 1987. 156(5): p. 1357.

195. Ente G, P.P., Kenisberg K, *Giant Umbilical Cord Associated With Patent Urachus. An External Clue to an Internal Anomaly.* Am J Dis Child, 1970. 120: p. 82.

196. Horn, L.C., et al., *Umbilical cord hypercoiling and thinning: a rare cause of intrauterine death in the second trimester of pregnancy.* Pediatr Dev Pathol, 2006. 9(1): p. 20-4.

197. Iwasaki, I., et al., *Isolated well-formed intestinal tissue in the umbilical cord. A variant of cyst of omphalomesenteric duct.* Acta Pathol Jpn, 1986. 36(4): p. 565-9.

198. Casola, G., W. Scheible, and G.R. Leopold, *Large umbilical cord: a normal finding in some fetuses.* Radiology, 1985. 156(1): p. 181-2.

199. Howorka, E. and W. Kapczynski, *Unusual thickness of the fetal end of the umbilical cord.* J Obstet Gynaecol Br Commonw, 1971. 78(3): p. 283.

200. Chantler, C., et al., *Giant umbilical cord associated with a patent urachus and fused umbilical arteries.* J Obstet Gynaecol Br Commonw, 1969. 76(3): p. 273-4.

201. Ogino, M., et al., *[Study on the histopathological abnormalities of the umbilical cord].* Nippon Sanka Fujinka Gakkai Zasshi, 1985. 37(3): p. 329-35.

202. Skulstad, S.M., et al., *The effect of umbilical venous constriction on placental development, cord length and perinatal outcome.* Early Hum Dev, 2005. 81(4): p. 325-31.

203. El Behery, M.M., et al., *Effect of umbilical vein blood flow on perinatal outcome of fetuses with lean and/or hypo-coiled umbilical cord.* Arch Gynecol Obstet, 2009.

204. Iffy, L. and V. Varadi, *Cerebral palsy following cutting of the nuchal cord before delivery.* Med Law, 1994. 13(3-4): p. 323-30.

205. Amiel-Tison, C.L. and A. Stewart, *The newborn infant; one brain for life.* 1994, INSERM; Paris, France.

206. Milovanov, A.P. and I.B. Glukhovets, *[Functional morphology of the neonatal umbilical cord during cesarean section].* Arkh Patol, 2007. 69(2): p. 28-30.

207. Raio, L., et al., *Hyaluronan content of Wharton's jelly in healthy and Down syndrome fetuses.* Matrix Biol, 2005. 24(2): p. 166-74.

208. Silver, R.K., et al., *Umbilical cord size and amniotic fluid volume in prolonged pregnancy.* Am J Obstet Gynecol, 1987. 157(3): p. 716-20.

209. Ali, A.F., et al., *Lack of proteoglycans in Wharton's jelly of the human umbilical cord as a cause of unexplained fetal loss in diabetic infants.* Obstet Gynecol, 2000. 95 (4 Suppl 1): p. S61-2.

210. Gill, P. and D. Jarjoura, *Wharton's jelly in the umbilical cord. A study of its quantitative variations and clinical correlates.* J Reprod Med, 1993. 38(8): p. 611-4.

211. Sloper, K.S., R.S. Brown, and J.D. Baum, *The water content of the human umbilical cord.* Early Hum Dev, 1979. 3(2): p. 205-10.

212. Meyer, F.A., *Wharton's jelly of the umbilical cord* Extracellular Matrix. Tissue Function, ed. W.D. Comper. Vol. 1. 1996, Amsterdam, Netherlands: Hardwood Academic Publishers.

213. Di Naro, E., et al., *Umbilical vein blood flow in fetuses with normal and lean umbilical cord.* Ultrasound Obstet Gynecol, 2001. 17(3): p. 224-8.

214. Di Naro, E., et al., *Umbilical cord morphology and pregnancy outcome.* Eur J Obstet Gynecol and Reprod Biol, 2001. 96: p. 150-157.

215. Strong, T.H., Jr., A.P. Sarno, and R.H. Paul, *Significance of intrapartum amniotic fluid volume in the presence of nuchal cords.* J Reprod Med, 1992. 37(8): p. 718-20.

216. Secco, M., et al., *Gene Expression Profile of Mesenchymal Stem Cells from Paired Umbilical Cord Units: Cord is Different from Blood.* Stem Cell Rev Rep, 2009.

217. Secco, M., et al., *Multipotent stem cells from umbilical cord: cord is richer than blood!* Stem Cells, 2008. 26(1): p. 146-50.

218. Wu, K.H., et al., *Cardiac potential of stem cells from whole human umbilical cord tissue.* J Cell Biochem, 2009. 107(5): p. 926-32.

219. Liu, M., et al., *[Comparative study of in vitro hematopoietic supportive capability of human mesenchymal stem cells derived from bone marrow and umbilical cord.].* Zhongguo Shi Yan Xue Ye Xue Za Zhi, 2009. 17(5): p. 1294-300.

220. Lu, L.L., et al., *Isolation and characterization of human umbilical cord mesenchymal stem cells with hematopoiesis-supportive function and other potentials.* Haematologica, 2006. 91(8): p. 1017-26.

221. Chen, M.Y., et al., *Endothelial differentiation of Wharton's jelly-derived mesenchymal stem cells in comparison with bone marrow-derived mesenchymal stem cells.* Exp Hematol, 2009. 37(5): p. 629-40.

222. Can, A. and S. Karahuseyinoglu, *Concise review: human umbilical cord stroma with regard to the source of fetus-derived stem cells.* Stem Cells, 2007. 25(11): p. 2886-95.

223. Rachakatla, R.S. and D. Troyer, *Wharton's jelly stromal cells as potential delivery vehicles for cancer therapeutics.* Future Oncol, 2009. 5(8): p. 1237-44.

224. Ayuzawa, R., et al., *Naive human umbilical cord matrix derived stem cells significantly attenuate growth of human breast cancer cells in vitro and in vivo.* Cancer Lett, 2009. 280(1): p. 31-7.

225. Weiss, M.L. and D.L. Troyer, *Stem cells in the umbilical cord.* Stem Cell Rev, 2006. 2(2): p. 155-62.

226. Breymann, C., D. Schmidt, and S.P. Hoerstrup, *Umbilical cord cells as a source of cardiovascular tissue engineering.* Stem Cell Rev, 2006. 2(2): p. 87-92.

227. Murai A., e.a., *Brief Communications and Case Reports: Umbilical Cord Teratoma in a Giraff.* Vet Pathol, 2007. 44: p. 204-206.

228. Stallabrass, P., *Long Cord.* British Med J, 1960. August: p. 603.

229. Berg, T.G. and W.F. Rayburn, *Umbilical cord length and acid-base balance at delivery.* J Reprod Med, 1995. 40(1): p. 9-12.

230. Krakowiak, P., et al., *Risk factors and outcomes associated with a short umbilical cord.* Obstet Gynecol, 2004. 103: p. 119-27.

231. Taweevisit, M. and P.S. Thorner, *'Massive' Fetal Thrombotic Vasculopathy Associated with Excessively Long Umbilical Cord in a Stillbirth: Case Report.* Pediatr Dev Pathol, 2009.

232. Izumi, K., et al., *Umbilical cord length in urinary tract abnormalities associated with oligohydramnios: evidence regarding developmental pathogenesis.* Fetal Pediatr Pathol, 2006. 25(5): p. 233-40.

233. Naeye, R.L., *Umbilical cord length: clinical significance.* J Pediatr, 1985. 107(2): p. 278-81.

234. Sarwono, E., et al., *Umbilical cord length and intra uterine wellbeing.* Paediatr Indones, 1991. 31(5-6): p. 136-40.

235. Wu, J.F., et al., *Multivariate analyses of the relationship between umbilical cord length and obstetric outcome.* Changgeng Yi Xue Za Zhi, 1996. 19(3): p. 247-52.

236. Rayburn, W.F., A. Beynen, and D.L. Brinkman, *Umbilical cord length and intrapartum complications.* Obstet Gynecol, 1981. 57(4): p. 450-2.

237. Hanley, L.C., T.K. Boyd, and J.L. Hecht, *Acardiac twin presenting as fetus amorphous with an attenuated umbilical cord.* Pediatr Dev Pathol, 2007. 10(6): p. 487-90.

238. Tycko, B., *Imprinted genes in placental growth and obstetric disorders.* Cytogenet Genome Res, 2006. 113(1-4): p. 271-8.

239. Craven, C.M., J.C. Carey, and K. Ward, *Umbilical cord agenesis in limb body wall defect.* Am J Med Genet, 1997. 71(1): p. 97-105.

240. Astner, A., et al., *Sonographically detected fetal and placental abnormalities associated with trisomy 16 confined to the placenta. A case report and review of the literature.* Prenat Diagn, 1998. 18(12): p. 1308-15.

241. Chan, Y., et al., *Maternal uniparental disomy of chromosome 16 and body stalk anomaly.* Am J Med Genet, 2000. 94(4): p. 284-6.

242. Ginsberg, N.E., A. Cadkin, and C. Strom, *Prenatal diagnosis of body stalk anomaly in the first trimester of pregnancy.* Ultrasound Obstet Gynecol, 1997. 10(6): p. 419-21.

243. Colpaert, C., et al., *Limb-body wall complex: 4 new cases illustrating the importance of examining placenta and umbilical cord.* Pathol Res Pract, 2000. 196(11): p. 783-90.

244. Daskalakis, G., et al., *Body stalk anomaly at 10-14 weeks of gestation.* Ultrasound Obstet Gynecol, 1997. 10(6): p. 416-8.

245. LaMonica, G., *Minimum cord length that allows spontaneous vaginal delivery.* J Reprod Med, 2008. 53(3): p. 217-9.

246. Sherer, D.M., et al., *Prenatal sonographic diagnosis of short umbilical cord in a dichorionic twin with normal fetal anatomy.* J Clin Ultrasound, 2009.

247. Mills, J.L., E.E. Harley, and A.C. Moessinger, *Standards for measuring umbilical cord length.* Placenta, 1983. 4(4): p. 423-6.

248. Miller, M.E., M.C. Jones, and D.W. Smith, *Tension: the basis of umbilical cord growth.* J Pediatr, 1982. 101(5): p. 844.

249. Fujinaga, M., A. Chinn, and T.H. Shepard, *Umbilical cord growth in human and rat fetuses: evidence against the "stretch hypothesis".* Teratology, 1990. 41(3): p. 333-9.

250. Moessinger, A.C., et al., *Umbilical cord length as an index of fetal activity: experimental study and clinical implications.* Pediatr Res, 1982. 16(2): p. 109-12.

251. Bohm, N., *[The missing umbilical cord syndrome--a typical malformation sequence].* Verh Dtsch Ges Pathol, 1982. 66: p. 436-9.

252. Giacoia, G.P., *Body stalk anomaly: congenital absence of the umbilical cord.* Obstet Gynecol, 1992. 80(3 Pt 2): p. 527-9.

253. Gilbert-Barness, E., et al., *Developmental abnormalities resulting in short umbilical cord.* Birth Defects Orig Artic Ser, 1993. 29(1): p. 113-40.

254. Sornes, T., *Short umbilical cord as a cause of fetal distress.* Acta Obstet Gynecol Scand, 1989. 68(7): p. 609-11.

255. Collins, J., *The short umbilical cord.* Am J Obstet Gynecol, 1992. 166(1 Pt 1): p. 268-9.

256. Bain, C. and B.W. Eliot, *Fetal Distress in the First Stage of Labour Associated with Early Fetal Heart Decelerations and*

a Short Umbilical Cord. Aust N Z J Obstet Gynaecol, 1976. 16: p. 51-56.

257. Flamm, B.L., *Tight nuchal cord and shoulder dystocia: a potentially catastrophic combination.* Obstet Gynecol, 1999. 94(5 Pt 2): p. 853.

258. Mantas, N., et al., *Intraabdominal umbilical vein dilatation and term delivery. A case report and review of the literature.* Fetal Diagn Ther, 2007. 22(6): p. 431-4.

259. Boue, D.R., C. Stanley, and R.N. Baergen, *Placental pathology casebook. Long umbilical cord with torsion and diffuse chorionic surface vein thrombosis: multiple associated congenital abnormalities including destructive encephalopathy.* J Perinatol, 1995. 15(5): p. 429-31.

260. Calvano, C.J., et al., *Experimental study of umbilical cord length as a marker of fetal alcohol syndrome.* Teratology, 2000. 61(3): p. 184-8.

261. Barron, S., E.P. Riley, and W.P. Smotherman, *The effect of prenatal alcohol exposure on umbilical cord length in fetal rats.* Alcohol Clin Exp Res, 1986. 10(5): p. 493-5.

262. Reynolds, S.R., et al., *The qualitative nature of pulsatile flow in umbilical blood vessels, with observations on flow in the aorta.* Bull Johns Hopkins Hosp, 1952. 91(2): p. 83-104.

263. Wright, J.W. and L.E. Ridgway, *Sources of variability in umbilical artery systolic/diastolic ratios: implications of the Poiseuille equation.* Am J Obstet Gynecol, 1990. 163(6 Pt 1): p. 1788-91.

264. Barron, S., J.A. Foss, and E.P. Riley, *The effect of prenatal cocaine exposure on umbilical cord length in fetal rats.* Neurotoxicol Teratol, 1991. 13(5): p. 503-6.

265. Durand, A., et al., *In utero measurement of the umbilical cord in full term pregnancy.* J Gynecol Obstet Biol Reprod, 1996. 25: p. 78-86.

266. De Silva, N., *Zygosity and umbilical cord length.* J Reprod Med, 1992. 37(10): p. 850-2.

267. Sornes, T. and T. Bakke, *Uterine size, parity and umbilical cord length.* Acta Obstet Gynecol Scand, 1989. 68(5): p. 439-41.

268. Soernes, T. and T. Bakke, *The length of the human umbilical cord in twin pregnancies.* Am J Obstet Gynecol, 1987. 157(5): p. 1229-30.

269. Soernes, T. and T. Bakke, *The length of the human umbilical cord in vertex and breech presentations.* Am J Obstet Gynecol, 1986. 154(5): p. 1086-7.

270. Hathout, H., *The Vascular Pattern and Mode of Insertion of the Umbilical Cord in Abortion Material.* J Obstet Gynaecol Br Commonw, 1964. 71: p. 963-4.

271. Perez-Cosio, C., E. Sheiner, and J.S. Abramowicz, *Four-vessel umbilical cord: not always a dire prognosis.* J Ultrasound Med, 2008. 27(9): p. 1389-91.

272. Bunce, D.F., 2nd, *Vascular arrangement in the umbilical cord.* J Am Osteopath Assoc, 1968. 67(9): p. 1010-2.

273. Larson, S.L., R.D. Kempers, and J.L. Titus, *Monoamniotic twins with a common umbilical cord.* Am J Obstet Gynecol, 1969. 105(4): p. 635-6.

274. Schimmel, M.S. and A.I. Eidelman, *Supernumerary umbilical vein resulting in a four-vessel umbilical cord.* Am J Perinatol, 1998. 15(5): p. 299-301.

275. Martinez, J.M., et al., *Biochemical and Doppler predictors of poor perinatal outcome in a fetus with four umbilical vessels.* Eur J Obstet Gynecol Reprod Biol, 1995. 62(1): p. 145-7.

276. Cohen, H.L., et al., *The multivessel umbilical cord: an antenatal indicator of possible conjoined twinning.* J Clin Ultrasound, 1992. 20(4): p. 278-82.

277. Beck, R. and C.M. Naulty, *A human umbilical cord with four arteries.* Clin Pediatr (Phila), 1985. 24(2): p. 118-9.

278. Painter, D. and P. Russell, *Four-vessel umbilical cord associated with multiple congenital anomalies.* Obstet Gynecol, 1977. 50(4): p. 505-7.

279. Murdoch, D.E., *Umbilical-cord doubling. Report of a case.* Obstet Gynecol, 1966. 27(4): p. 555-7.

280. Meyer, W.W., J. Lind, and M. Moinian, *An accessory fourth vessel of the umbilical cord. A preliminary study.* Am J Obstet Gynecol, 1969. 105(7): p. 1063-8.

281. Aoki, S., et al., *Antenatal diagnosis of aberrant umbilical vessels.* Gynecol Obstet Invest, 1997. 43(4): p. 232-5.

282. Pavlopoulos, P.M., et al., *Association of single umbilical artery with congenital malformations of vascular etiology.* Pediatr Dev Pathol, 1998. 1(6): p. 487-93.

283. Bjoro, K., Jr., *Vascular anomalies of the umbilical cord: I. Obstetric implications.* Early Hum Dev, 1983. 8(2): p. 119-27.

284. Csecsei, K., et al., *Incidence and associations of single umbilical artery in prenatally diagnosed malformed, midtrimester fetuses: a review of 62 cases.* Am J Med Genet, 1992. 43(3): p. 524-30.

285. Saller, D.N., Jr. and R. Neiger, *Cytogenetic abnormalities among perinatal deaths demonstrating a single umbilical artery.* Prenat Diagn, 1994. 14(1): p. 13-6.

286. Scalercio, F., et al., *[Single umbilical artery (SUA) and congenital eye abnormalities. 2 case reports].* Minerva Pediatr, 1998. 50(4): p. 141-4.

287. Hadar, A. and M. Hallak, *Single umbilical artery and umbilical cord torsion leading to fetal death. A case report.* J Reprod Med, 2003. 48(9): p. 739-40.

288. Dane, B., et al., *Fetuses with single umbilical artery: analysis of 45 cases.* Clin Exp Obstet Gynecol, 2009. 36(2): p. 116-9.

289. Mu, S.C., et al., *The perinatal outcomes of asymptomatic isolated single umbilical artery in full-term neonates.* Pediatr Neonatol, 2008. 49(6): p. 230-3.

290. Thummala, M.R., T.N. Raju, and P. Langenberg, *Isolated single umbilical artery anomaly and the risk for congenital malformations: a meta-analysis.* J Pediatr Surg, 1998. 33(4): p. 580-5.

291. Visnovsky, J., et al., *[Single umbilical artery syndrome (review and a case report)].* Ceska Gynekol, 2008. 73(4): p. 250-3.

292. Martinez-Frias, M.L., et al., *Does single umbilical artery (SUA) predict any type of congenital defect? Clinical-epidemiological analysis of a large consecutive series of malformed infants.* Am J Med Genet A, 2008. 146A(1): p. 15-25.

293. Nicolaides, K.H. and P. Wegrzyn, *[Sonographic features of chromosomal defects at 11(+0) to 13(+6) weeks of gestation].* Ginekol Pol, 2005. 76(6): p. 423-30.

294. Catanzarite, V., M. Jones, and C. Maida, *The two-vessel cord: How concerned should we be.* Contemporary OB/GYN, 1997. April: p. 43-54.

295. Sepulveda, W., et al., *Discordant iliac and femoral artery flow velocity waveforms in fetuses with single umbilical artery.* Am J Obstet Gynecol, 1994. 171(2): p. 521-5.

296. Persutte, W.H. and R.R. Lenke, *Transverse umbilical arterial diameter: technique for the prenatal diagnosis of single umbilical artery.* J Ultrasound Med, 1994. 13(10): p. 763-6.

297. Abuhamad, A.Z., et al., *Single umbilical artery: does it matter which artery is missing?* Am J Obstet Gynecol, 1995. 173(3 Pt 1): p. 728-32.

298. Ulm, B., et al., *Umbilical artery Doppler velocimetry in fetuses with a single umbilical artery.* Obstet Gynecol, 1997. 90(2): p. 205-9.

299. Fukada, Y., T. Yasumizu, and K. Hoshi, *Single umbilical artery: correlation of the prognosis and side of the missing artery.* Int J Gynaecol Obstet, 1998. 61(1): p. 67-8.

300. Geipel, A., et al., *Prenatal diagnosis of single umbilical artery: determination of the absent side, associated anomalies, Doppler findings and perinatal outcome.* Ultrasound Obstet Gynecol, 2000. 15(2): p. 114-7.

301. Rinehart, B.K., et al., *Single umbilical artery is associated with an increased incidence of structural and chromosomal anomalies and growth restriction.* Am J Perinatol, 2000. 17(5): p. 229-32.

302. Pierce, B.T., et al., *Perinatal outcome following fetal single umbilical artery diagnosis.* J Matern Fetal Med, 2001. 10(1): p. 59-63.

303. Tarnier, E.S. and G. Chantreuil, *Traite de l'art des Accouchements*, 1882; Paris, France. Pg 393.

304. Chaurasia, B.D. and B.M. Agarwal, *Helical structure of the human umbilical cord.* Acta Anat (Basel), 1979. 103(2): p. 226-30.

305. Fletcher, S., *Chirality in the umbilical cord.* Br J Obstet Gynaecol, 1993. 100(3): p. 234-6.

306. Ochshorn, Y., et al., *Coiling characteristics of umbilical cords in breech vs. vertex presentation.* J Perinat Med, 2009. 37(5): p. 525-8.

307. Vizza, E., et al., *The collagen skeleton of the human umbilical cord at term. A scanning electron microscopy study after 2N-NaOH maceration.* Reprod Fertil Dev, 1996. 8(5): p. 885-94.

308. Salvolini, E., et al., *Growth retardation and discordant twin pregnancy. An immunomorphological and biochemical characterisation of the human umbilical cord.* Biochem Mol Biol Int, 1998. 46(4): p. 795-805.

309. Hofstaetter, C., M. Dubiel, and S. Gudmundsson, *Two types of umbilical venous pulsations and outcome of high-risk pregnancy.* Early Hum Dev, 2001. 61(2): p. 111-7.

310. S Sunagawa, e.a., *Nonimmunologic hydrops fetalis associated with polypoid embolizations of both embolizations.* Prenatal Diagnosis, 2008. 28(8): p. 776-7.

311. Baxi, L.V., A. Daftary, and A. Loucopoulos, *Single fetal demise in a twin gestation: umbilical vein thrombosis.* Gynecol Obstet Invest, 1998. 46(4): p. 266-7.

312. Bagyanszki, M., et al., *Structural differences in the umbilical vein wall after full-term and pre-term delivery.* Anat Histol Embryol, 2009. 38(5): p. 387-91.

313. Decastel, M., et al., *Morphological features of the human umbilical vein in normal, sickle cell trait, and sickle cell disease pregnancies.* Hum Pathol, 1999. 30(1): p. 13-20.

314. Stehbens, W.E., et al., *Histopathology and ultrastructure of human umbilical blood vessels.* Fetal Pediatr Pathol, 2005. 24(6): p. 297-315.

315. Hoang-Ngoc, M., et al., *[Structure and function of the fetal umbilical vessels].* J Gynecol Obstet Biol Reprod (Paris), 1985. 14(8): p. 973-9.

316. Sexton, A.J., et al., *A study of the ultrastructure of developing human umbilical vessels.* J Anat, 1996. 188 (Pt 1): p. 75-85.

317. McGuigan, A.P. and M.V. Sefton, *The thrombogenicity of human umbilical vein endothelial cell seeded collagen modules.* Biomaterials, 2008. 29(16): p. 2453-63.

318. Atalla, R.K., et al., *Newborn acid-base status and umbilical cord morphology.* Obstet Gynecol, 1998. 92(5): p. 865-8.

319. Barr, M., Jr., *Organ asymmetries as correlates of other anomalies.* Am J Med Genet, 2001. 101(4): p. 328-33.

320. Collins, J.H., *Discordant umbilical cord structure in a twin gestation.* J Ultrasound Med, 1994. 13(10): p. 742.

321. Collins, J.H., *A photographic look at umbilical cord vessel variation.* Am J Obstet Gynecol, 1995. 172(2 Pt 1): p. 718-20.

322. Dado, G.M., P.B. Dobrin, and R.S. Mrkvicka, *Venous flow through coiled and noncoiled umbilical cords. Effects of*

external compression, twisting and longitudinal stretching. J Reprod Med, 1997. 42(9): p. 576-80.

323. Jakobovits, A., *[Non-coiled umbilical cord as a potential risk factor to the fetus].* Orv Hetil, 1996. 137(38): p. 2081-2.

324. Machin, G.A., J. Ackerman, and E. Gilbert-Barness, *Abnormal umbilical cord coiling is associated with adverse perinatal outcomes.* Pediatr Dev Pathol, 2000. 3(5): p. 462-71.

325. Nakai, Y., et al., *Umbilical venous pulsation associated with hypercoiled cord in growth-retarded fetuses.* Gynecol Obstet Invest, 1997. 43(1): p. 64-7.

326. Pande, B.S. and I. Singh, *One-sided dominance in the upper limbs of human fetuses as evidenced by asymmetry in muscle and bone weight.* J Anat, 1971. 109(Pt 3): p. 457-9.

327. Petrikovsky, B. and B. Gross, *Umbilical cord: coiled versus noncoiled--is there a third variant?* J Clin Ultrasound, 1996. 24(6): p. 321-2.

328. Predanic, M., et al., *Disparate blood flow patterns in parallel umbilical arteries.* Obstet Gynecol, 1998. 91(5 Pt 1): p. 757-60.

329. Sonesson, S.E., et al., *Reference values for Doppler velocimetric indices from the fetal and placental ends of the umbilical artery during normal pregnancy.* J Clin Ultrasound, 1993. 21(5): p. 317-24.

330. Strong, T.H., Jr., J.P. Elliott, and T.G. Radin, *Non-coiled umbilical blood vessels: a new marker for the fetus at risk.* Obstet Gynecol, 1993. 81(3): p. 409-11.

331. Tan, U. and N. Zor, *Grasp-reflex strength from right and left hands in relation to serum cortisol level and fetal position in human neonates.* Int J Neurosci, 1994. 74(1-4): p. 27-32.

332. Cullen, T.S., *Embryology, Anatomy and Diseases of the Umbilicus*, 1916, W B Saunders. Philadelphia, PA.

333. Hasegawa, J., et al., *Cord insertion into the lower third of the uterus in the first trimester is associated with placental and umbilical cord abonormalities.* Ultrasound Obstet Gynecol, 2006. 28(2): p. 183-6.

334. Lurie, S., K. Fenakel, and S. Gorbacz, *Antenatal maceration of umbilical cord; a case report.* Eur J Obstet Gynecol Reprod Biol, 1990. 35(2-3): p. 271-4.

335. Kamitomo, M., et al., *Hemangioma of the umbilical cord: stenotic change of the umbilical vessels.* Fetal Diagn Ther, 1999. 14(6): p. 328-31.

336. Dougall, A. and C.H. Baird, *Vasa praevia--report of three cases and review of literature.* Br J Obstet Gynaecol, 1987. 94(7): p. 712-5.

337. Fujiyama, T., R. Yamaguchi, and K. Noda, *Nerve distribution in human fetal appendages, particularly in the umbilical cord.* Tohoku J Exp Med, 1971. 105(2): p. 111-21.

338. Jutte, J.J., H.G. Geerdink, and B. Baljet, *The innervation of the umbilical cord of the rat. A histochemical study.* Acta Morphol Neerl Scand, 1977. 15(2): p. 135-41.

339. Walker, D.W. and J.R. McLean, *Absence of adrenergic nerves in the human placenta.* Nature, 1971. 229(5283): p. 344-5.

340. Anthonioz, P. and M. Maillet, *[Demonstration of an innervation in the umbilical cord in rats].* C R Seances Soc Biol Fil, 1972. 166(10): p. 1250-3.

341. Aburel, E., et al., *Innervation des Mutterkuchens, der Nabelschnur und der intra-abdominalen Nabelgetafse des feten.* Obstet et Ginec, 1958. 6: p. 493.

342. Kilavuz, O. and K. Vetter, *The umbilical ring--the first rapid in the fetoplacental venous system.* J Perinat Med, 1998. 26(2): p. 120-2.

343. Skulstad, S.M., et al., *The development of high venous velocity at the fetal umbilical ring during gestational weeks 11-19.* BJOG, 2001. 108(3): p. 248-53.

344. Pearson, A.A. and R.W. Sauter, *The innervation of the umbilical vein in human embryos and fetuses.* Am J Anat, 1969. 125(3): p. 345-52.

345. Pearson, A.A. and R.W. Sauter, *Nerve contributions to the pelvic plexus and the umbilical cord.* Am J Anat, 1970. 128(4): p. 485-98.

346. Reilly, R.D. and P.T. Russell, *Neurohistochemical evidence supporting an absence of adrenergic and cholinergic innervation in the human placenta and umbilical cord.* Anat Rec, 1977. 188(3): p. 277-86.

347. Fox, S.B. and T.Y. Khong, *Lack of innervation of human umbilical cord. An immunohistological and histochemical study.* Placenta, 1990. 11(1): p. 59-62.

348. Kawano, M. and N. Mori, *[Confirmation of the presence of adrenergic fibers in human umbilical cord by electron microscopy].* Nippon Sanka Fujinka Gakkai Zasshi, 1989. 41(7): p. 833-6.

349. Jauniaux, E., et al., *Embryonic remnants of the umbilical cord: morphologic and clinical aspects.* Hum Pathol, 1989. 20(5): p. 458-62.

350. Heifetz SA, R.-P.M., *Omphalomesenteric duct cysts of the umbilical cord.* Pediatr Pathol, 1983. 1: p. 325.

351. Jauniaux E, D.C., Thomas C, et al, *Umbilical Cord Pseudocyst in Trisomy 18.* Prenat Diagn, 1988. 8: p. 557.

352. Kuwata T, M.s., Izumi,et al., *Umbilical cord pseudocyst in a fetus with trisomy 18.* Fetal Diagn Ther, 2003. 18(8).

353. Ross JA, J.D., ZoZosmer N, et al, *Umbilical Cord Cyst in Early Pregnancy* Obstet Gynecol, 1997. 89: p. 442.

354. Howarka E, K.W., *Unusual thickness of the fetal end of the umbilical cord.* J Obstet Gynaecol Br Commonw, 1971. 78: p. 283.

355. Kita, M., et al., *Umbilical Cord Cysts of Allantoic and Omphalomesenteric Remnants with Progressive Umbilical Cord Edema: A Case Report.* Fetal Diagn Ther, 2009. 25(2): p. 250-254.

356. Fuchs, F., et al., *Prenatal diagnosis of a patent urachus cyst with the use of 2D, 3D, 4D ultrasound and fetal magnetic resonance imaging.* Fetal Diagn Ther, 2008. 24(4): p. 444-7.

357. Rempen, A., *Sonographic first-trimester diagnosis of umbilical cord cyst.* J Clin Ultrasound, 1989. 17(1): p. 53-5.

358. Zelante, L. and B. Dallapiccola, *Umbilical cord pseudocyst in trisomy 13.* Prenat Diagn, 1989. 9(6): p. 448-9.

359. Yonemoto, H., et al., *Umbilical cord cyst detected in the first trimester by two- and three-dimensional sonography.* J Clin Ultrasound, 2006. 34(3): p. 150-2.

360. Bunch, P.T., et al., *Allantoic cyst: a prenatal clue to patent urachus.* Pediatr Radiol, 2006. 36(10): p. 1090-5.

361. Alimoglu, E., et al., *Umbilical cord pseudocyst in a fetus with Down syndrome.* Prenat Diagn, 2006. 26(2): p. 193-4.

362. Smith, G.N., et al., *The sonographic finding of persistent umbilical cord cystic masses is associated with lethal aneuploidy and/or congenital anomalies.* Prenat Diagn, 1996. 16(12): p. 1141-7.

363. Guschmann, M., et al., *[Intestinal polyp of the umbilical cord].* Zentralbl Gynakol, 2002. 124(2): p. 132-4.

364. Ghezzi, F., et al., *Single and multiple umbilical cord cysts in early gestation: two different entities.* Ultrasound Obstet Gynecol, 2003. 21(3): p. 215-9.

365. O'Marcaigh, A.S., L.B. Folz, and V.V. Michels, *Umbilical morphology: normal values for neonatal periumbilical skin length.* Pediatrics, 1992. 90(1 Pt 1): p. 47-9.

366. Oyelese, Y., et al., *Magnetic resonance imaging of vasa praevia.* BJOG, 2003. 110(12): p. 1127-8.

367. Nimmo, M.J., D. Kinsella, and H.S. Andrews, *MRI in pregnancy: the diagnosis of vasa previa by magnetic resonance imaging.* Bristol Med Chir J, 1988. 103(2): p. 12.

368. Pretorius, D.H., et al., *Placental cord insertion visualization with prenatal ultrasonography.* J Ultrasound Med, 1996. 15(8): p. 585-93.

369. Wilson, B., *Sonography of the placenta and umbilical cord.* Radiologic Technology, 2008. 79(4): p. 333S-345S.

370. Gagnon, R., et al., *Guidelines for the management of vasa previa.* J Obstet Gynaecol Can, 2009. 31(8): p. 748-60.

371. Sinha, P., et al., *Vasa praevia: a missed diagnosis.* J Obstet Gynaecol, 2008. 28(6): p. 600-3.

372. Tang, M.Y., *[Pathologic analysis of the placenta in preterm deliveries]*. Zhonghua Fu Chan Ke Za Zhi, 1989. 24(6): p. 334-7, 380-1.

373. Robinson, L.K., K.L. Jones, and K. Benirschke, *The nature of structural defects associated with velamentous and marginal insertion of the umbilical cord*. Am J Obstet Gynecol, 1983. 146(2): p. 191-3.

374. Peng, H.Q., et al., *Umbilical cord stricture and overcoiling are common causes of fetal demise*. Pediatr Dev Pathol, 2006. 9(1): p. 14-9.

375. Sun, Y., et al., *Umbilical cord stricture and intrauterine fetal death*. Pediatr Pathol Lab Med, 1995. 15(5): p. 723-32.

376. Weber, J., *Constriction of the Umbilical Cord as a Cause of Foetal Death*. Acta Obstet Gynecol Scand, 1963. 42: p. 259-68.

377. Van Vugt, P.J.H., *De betekenis van het verloop van de bloedvaten in de navelstreng*. Vergadering, 1968. 16: p. 127-138.

378. Ontiveros Lira, D., et al., *[Umbilical cord stenosis and nonimmunological hydrops fetalis. A case report]*. Ginecol Obstet Mex, 1988. 56: p. 277-80.

379. Meir, K., et al., *Single umbilical artery stenosis associated with intrauterine fetal death post-transfusion*. Prenat Diagn, 2002. 22(3): p. 186-8.

380. Burton, G. and D.M. Saunders, *Vasa praevia: another cause for concern in in vitro fertilization pregnancies*. Aust N Z J Obstet Gynaecol, 1988. 28(3): p. 180-1.

381. Vestermark, K.V., et al., *Spontaneous intra-uterine total rupture of a velamentous umbilical cord; a case report.* Eur J Obstet Gynecol 1989. 35: p. 279-81.

382. Woods, D.L. and A.F. Malan, *The site of umbilical cord insertion and birth weight.* Br J Obstet Gynaecol, 1978. 85(5): p. 332-3.

383. Nordenvall, M., B. Sandstedt, and U. Ulmsten, *Relationship between placental shape, cord insertion, lobes and gestational outcome.* Acta Obstet Gynecol Scand, 1988. 67(7): p. 611-6.

384. Kouyoumdjian, A., *Velamentous insertion of the umbilical cord.* Obstet Gynecol, 1980. 56(6): p. 737-42.

385. Fung, T.Y. and T.K. Lau, *Poor perinatal outcome associated with vasa previa: is it preventable? A report of three cases and review of the literature.* Ultrasound Obstet Gynecol, 1998. 12(6): p. 430-3.

386. Heinonen, S., et al., *Perinatal diagnostic evaluation of velamentous umbilical cord insertion: clinical, Doppler, and ultrasonic findings.* Obstet Gynecol, 1996. 87(1): p. 112-7.

387. Jaovisidha, A. and Y. Herabutya, *Vasa previa in Ramathibodi Hospital: a 10 years review.* J Med Assoc Thai, 1998. 81(12): p. 998-1002.

388. Yi, T.M., *Pathologic analysis of preterm delivery placentas.* Chin Med J, 1990. 103: p. 856-861.

389. Monie, I.W., *Velamentous Insertion of the Cord in Early Pregnancy.* Am J Obstet Gynecol, 1965. 93: p. 276-81.

390. Collins, J.H., *First report: telemetry-assisted ambulatory nonstress test to evaluate umbilical cord compression.* Am J Obstet Gynecol, 1992. 166(3): p. 1020-1.

391. Loos, R.J., et al., *Birthweight in liveborn twins: the influence of the umbilical cord insertion and fusion of placentas.* BJOG, 2001. 108(9): p. 943-8.

392. Clark, J.F., *Fetal heart monitoring in detection velamentous insertion of the umbilical cord.* J Natl Med Assoc, 1984. 76(3): p. 292-4.

393. Kitsunezuka, S., *[Sites of placental attachment to the uterus and the umbilical cord attachment at the uterine periphery].* Josanpu Zasshi, 1974. 28(12): p. 652-5.

394. Otsubo, Y., et al., *Sonographic evaluation of umbilical cord insertion with umbilical coiling index.* J Clin Ultrasound, 1999. 27(6): p. 341-4.

395. Fries, M.H., et al., *The role of velamentous cord insertion in the etiology of twin-twin transfusion syndrome.* Obstet Gynecol, 1993. 81(4): p. 569-74.

396. Craven, F.O.K., *Neonatal Death due to Litigation of Umbilical Cord by an Amniotic Band.* British Medical Journal, 1953(Jan 10th): p. 81.

397. Editorial, *Amniotic Bands.* British Medical Journal, 1973(Sept 29): p. 651-652.

398. Sifakis, S., et al., *A stillborn fetus with amniotic band syndrome and elevated levels of alpha-fetoprotein plus beta-human chorionic gonadotropin: a case report.* Fetal Diagn Ther, 2008. 24(2): p. 111-4.

399. Heifetz, S.A., *Strangulation of the umbilical cord by amniotic bands: report of 6 cases and literature review.* Pediatr Pathol, 1984. 2(3): p. 285-304.

400. Lurie, S., M. Feinstein, and Y. Mamet, *Umbilical cord strangulation by an amniotic band resulting in a stillbirth.* J Obstet Gynaecol Res, 2008. 34(2): p. 255-7.

401. Elchalal, U., et al., *Strangulation of the umbilical cord due to combined amniotic band and true knot.* Int J Gynaecol Obstet, 1992. 38(1): p. 45-7.

402. Voss, M.K., L.S. Hansen, and K.L. Rasmussen, *[Umbilical cord constriction caused by amniotic band].* Ugeskr Laeger, 2007. 169(41): p. 3497-8.

403. Strauss, A., et al., *Intra-uterine fetal demise caused by amniotic band syndrome after standard amniocentesis.* Fetal Diagn Ther, 2000. 15(1): p. 4-7.

404. Reles, A., et al., *[Intrauterine fetal death after strangulation of the umbilical cord by amniotic bands].* Geburtshilfe Frauenheilkd, 1991. 51(12): p. 1006-8.

405. Husler, M.R., et al., *When is fetoscopic release of amniotic bands indicated? Review of outcome of cases treated in utero and selection criteria for fetal surgery.* Prenat Diagn, 2009. 29(5): p. 457-63.

406. Moran, S.L., M. Jensen, and C. Bravo, *Amniotic band syndrome of the upper extremity: diagnosis and management.* J Am Acad Orthop Surg, 2007. 15(7): p. 397-407.

407. Sentilhes, L., et al., *[Amniotic band syndrome: pathogenesis, prenatal diagnosis and neonatal management].* J Gynecol Obstet Biol Reprod (Paris), 2003. 32(8 Pt 1): p. 693-704.

408. Peiro, J.L., et al., *Fetoscopic release of umbilical cord amniotic band in a human fetus.* Ultrasound Obstet Gynecol, 2009. 33(2): p. 232-4.

409. Inubashiri, E., et al., *3D and 4D sonographic imaging of amniotic band syndrome in early pregnancy.* J Clin Ultrasound, 2008. 36(9): p. 573-5.

410. Khong, T.Y., *Calcification of umbilical artery:two distinct lesions.* J Clin Pathology, 1989. 42: p. 931-934.

411. Mc Millan, H.M., et al., *Combination of vasa praevia, true umbilical cord knot and a subserosal hemorrhage.* J Perinat Med, 2006. 34(1): p. 88.

412. Karin, P., et al. *Diagnostic evaluation of intrauterine fetal deaths in Stockholm 1998-99.* Acta Obstet Gynecol Scand, 2002. 81: p. 284-92.

413. Cunningham, F.G. and L.M. Hollier, *Fetal Death (Supplement).* Williams Obstetrics (ed 20), ed. F.G. Cunningham, et al., 1997; Simon & Schuster, N.Y., N.Y.

414. Hofmeyr, G.J. and A.M. Gulmezoglu, *Maternal hydration for increasing amniotic fluid volume in oligohydramnios and normal amniotic fluid volume.* Cochrane Database Syst Rev, 2002(1): p. CD000134.

415. *Fetal Growth Disorders.* Williams Obstetrics (ed 21), ed. F.G. Cunningham, et al., McGraw-Hill; N.Y., N.Y. 2001: 746.

416. Tan, S.J., et al., *Fetal demise by umbilical cord around abdomen and stricture.* Arch Gynecol Obstet, 2009.

417. Poljak, B., et al., *[Prenatal diagnosis of coiling of the umbilical cord around the neck and its effect on early neonatal prognosis].* Lijec Vjesn, 1989. 111(8): p. 260-2.

418. Carp, H.J., ed. *Recurrent Pregnancy Loss ; Causes, Controversies and Treatment.* Series in Maternal Fetal Medicine. 2007, Informa Healthcare: NY. 73.

419. Glanfield, P.A. and R. Watson, *Intrauterine fetal death due to umbilical cord torsion.* Arch Pathol Lab Med, 1986. 110(4): p. 357-8.

420. Ben-Arie, A., et al., *Oligohydramnios, intrauterine growth retardation and fetal death due to umbilical cord torsion.* Arch Gynecol Obstet, 1995. 256(3): p. 159-61.

421. Utsu, M. and K. Maeda, *Distinction of the pahologic hyper-torsion from the physiological spiral development of the umbilical cord.* Choonpa Igaku Jap J Med Ultrasonics, 1991. 18: p. 607-608.

422. Fleisch, M.C. and T. Hoehn, *Intrauterine fetal death after multiple umbilical cord torsion-complication of a twin pregnancy following assisted reproduction.* J Assist Reprod Genet, 2008. 25(6): p. 277-9.

423. Bendon, R.W., *Articles on umbilical cord torsion and fetal death.* Pediatr Dev Pathol, 2007. 10(2): p. 165-6.

424. Herman, A., et al., *Extremely large number of twists of the umbilical cord causing torsion and intrauterine fetal death.* Int J Gynaecol Obstet, 1991. 35(2): p. 165-7.

425. Frazer., G.S., *Umbilical Cord compromise as a cause of abortion.* Equine Veterinary Education, 2007(November): p. 535-537.

426. Hong, C.B., et al., *Equine abortion and stillbirth in central Kentucky during 1988 and 1989 foaling seasons.* J Vet Diagn Invest, 1993. 5(4): p. 560-6.

427. Smith, K.C., et al., *A survey of equine abortion, stillbirth and neonatal death in the UK from 1988 to 1997.* Equine Vet J, 2003. 35(5): p. 496-501.

428. Gurung, G. and A. Rana, *Extensive torsion of umbilical cord: a rare cause of fetal compromise.* Nepal Med Coll J, 2006. 8(1): p. 61-2.

429. Vandeplassche, M. and H. Lauwers, *The twisted umbilical cord: an expression of kinesis of the equine fetus.* Animal Reproduction Science, 1986. 10: p. 163-175.

430. Roberts, S.J., *Abortion and other diseases of gestation in mares.* Current Therapy in Theriogenology, ed. D.W. Morrow, W B Saunders, Philadelphia, PA, 1287.

431. Kaplan, A., *Hemodynamic analysis of arterial blood flow in the coiled umbilical cord.* Reprod Sci, 2010. 17(3): p. 258-68.

432. Lacro, R.V., K.L. Jones, and K. Benirschke, *The umbilical cord twist: origin, direction, and relevance.* Am J Obstet Gynecol, 1987. 157(4 Pt 1): p. 833-8.

433. Edmonds, H.W., *The spiral twist of the normal umbilical cord in twins and in singletons.* Am J Obstet Gynecol, 1954. 67(1): p. 102-20.

434. Tian, C.F., et al., *Relationship between pitch value or S/D ratio of torsion of cord and fetal outcome.* Prenat Diagn. 30(5): p. 454-8.

435. Zhou, C.J., *Fetal distress caused by umbilical cord anomalies; analysis of 456 cases.* J Practical Obstet Gynecol, 1990. 6: p. 316-17.

436. Zhao, L.T., *Extremely twisted cord and fetal death.* Chinese J Obstet Gynecol, 1964. 10(401-3).

437. Malpas, P. and E.M. Symonds, *Observations on the structure of the human umbilical cord.* Surg Gynecol Obstet, 1966. 123(4): p. 746-50.

438. de Laat, M.W., et al., *The umbilical coiling index, a review of the literature.* J Matern Fetal Neonatal Med, 2005. 17(2): p. 93-100.

439. Strong, T.H., Jr., et al., *The umbilical coiling index.* Am J Obstet Gynecol, 1994. 170(1 Pt 1): p. 29-32.

440. Ercal, T., et al., *Umbilical coiling index: is it a marker for the foetus at risk?* Br J Clin Pract, 1996. 50(5): p. 254-6.

441. Colgan, T.J. and S.C. Luk, *Umbilical-cord torsion, thrombosis, and intrauterine death of a twin fetus.* Arch Pathol Lab Med, 1982. 106(2): p. 101.

442. Virgilio, L.A. and D.B. Spangler, *Fetal death secondary to constriction and torsion of the umbilical cord.* Arch Pathol Lab Med, 1978. 102(1): p. 32-3.

443. Gilbert, E.F. and F.T. Zugibe, *Torsion and constriction of the umbilical cord. A cause of fetal death.* Arch Pathol, 1974. 97(1): p. 58-9.

444. Morparia, H., *Sonographic detection of umbilical cord twist.* J Ultrasound Med, 1993. 12(8): p. 471-2.

445. Cromi, A., et al., *Sonographic umbilical cord morphometry and coiling patterns in twin-twin transfusion syndrome.* Prenat Diagn, 2005. 25(9): p. 851-5.

446. Tang, M.Y., *The Pathology of the Placenta.* 1987, pg 42, Beijing, China: Peoples Health Publishing House.

447. Chang, D.Y., et al., *Triplet pregnancy complicated by intrauterine fetal death of conjoined twins from an umbilical cord accident of an acardius. A case report.* J Reprod Med, 1996. 41(6): p. 459-62.

448. Crawford, J.S., *Cord round the neck. Incidence and sequelae.* Acta Paediatr, 1962. 51: p. 594-603.

449. Kizer, S. and O. Aguero, *Circulares Del Cordon.* Revista de Obstet Gynecol de Venezuela, 1969. 29(85-95).

450. Collins, J.H., et al., *Nuchal cord: a definition and a study associating placental location and nuchal cord incidence.* J La State Med Soc, 1991. 143(7): p. 18-23.

451. Judy, C. and L.A. Bell, *A case of seven nuchal loops and a review of the literature.* Mo Med, 2005. 102(6): p. 569-70.

452. Wang, Y., et al., *Management of nuchal cord with multiple loops.* Obstet Gynecol, 2008. 112(2 Pt 2): p. 460-1.

453. Dursun, P., et al., *Nuchal cord type B associated with an excessively long umbilical cord as a cause of stillbirth: a case report.* Clin Exp Obstet Gynecol, 2004. 31(2): p. 158-9.

454. Giacomello, F., *Ultrasound determination of nuchal cord in breech presentation.* Am J Obstet Gynecol, 1987. 156: p. 531-32.

455. Collins, J.H., *Nuchal cord type A and type B.* Am J Obstet Gynecol, 1997. 177(1): p. 94.

456. Sherer, D.M., et al., *Is fetal cerebral vascular resistance affected by the presence of nuchal cord(s) in the third trimester of pregnancy?* Ultrasound Obstet Gynecol, 2005. 25(5): p. 454-8.

457. Xu, H., et al., *[Prediction of fetal hypoxia by measuring middle cerebral and umbilical artery resistance index in fetuses with umbilical cord around the neck in late pregnancy].* Nan Fang Yi Ke Da Xue Xue Bao, 2008. 28(12): p. 2207-9.

458. Szymanski, M., et al., *[Relationship between doppler velocimetry at middle cerebral artery and umbilical artery and status of newborn after delivery]*. Ginekol Pol, 2005. 76(9): p. 713-9.

459. Onan, A., et al., *Lipid peroxidation in nuchal cord cases: implication for fetal distress.* J Matern Fetal Neonatal Med, 2009. 22(3): p. 254-8.

460. Perlitz, Y., I. Ben-Shlomo, and M. Ben-Ami, *Acute polyhydramnios in term pregnancy may be caused by multiple nuchal cord loops.* Ultrasound Obstet Gynecol. 35(2): p. 253-254.

461. Onderoglu, L.S., P. Dursun, and T. Durukan, *Perinatal features and umbilical cord blood gases in newborns complicated with nuchal cord.* Turk J Pediatr, 2008. 50(5): p. 466-70.

462. Shrestha, N.S. and N. Singh, *Nuchal cord and perinatal outcome.* Kathmandu Univ Med J (KUMJ), 2007. 5(3): p. 360-3.

463. Sheiner, E., et al., *Nuchal cord is not associated with adverse perinatal outcome.* Arch Gynecol Obstet, 2006. 274(2): p. 81-3.

464. Assimakopoulos, E., et al., *Nuchal cord detected by ultrasound at term is associated with mode of delivery and perinatal outcome.* Eur J Obstet Gynecol Reprod Biol, 2005. 123(2): p. 188-92.

465. Schaffer, L., et al., *Nuchal cords in term and postterm deliveries--do we need to know?* Obstet Gynecol, 2005. 106(1): p. 23-8.

466. Rogers, M.S., et al., *Relationship between umbilical cord morphology and nuchal cord entanglement.* Acta Obstet Gynecol Scand, 2003. 82(1): p. 32-7.

467. Romero-Gutierrez, G., et al., *Multivariate analysis of risk factors for stillbirth in Leon, Mexico.* Acta Obstet Gynecol Scand, 2005. 84(1): p. 2-6.

468. Ogueh, O., et al., *Obstetrical factors related to nuchal cord.* Acta Obstet Gynecol Scand, 2006. 85(7): p. 810-4.

469. Abdu, A.T., et al., *Adrenal hemorrhage in a newborn.* Am J Perinatol, 2009. 26(8): p. 553-7.

470. Hasegawa, J., et al., *Ultrasound diagnosis and management of umbilical cord abnormalities.* Taiwan J Obstet Gynecol, 2009. 48(1): p. 23-7.

471. Tepper, R., et al., *High incidence of cord entanglement during early pregnancy detected by three-dimensional sonography.* Am J Perinatol, 2009. 26(5): p. 379-82.

472. Lal, N., D. Deka, and S. Mittal, *Does the nuchal cord persist? An ultrasound and color-Doppler-based prospective study.* J Obstet Gynaecol Res, 2008. 34(3): p. 314-7.

473. Jarvenpaa, J., et al., *Cord compression may rapidly influence the expression of placental angiogenic genes in pre-eclampsia.* Placenta, 2008. 29(5): p. 436-8.

474. Folkerth, R.D., et al., *Neuronal cell death in the arcuate nucleus of the medulla oblongata in stillbirth.* Int J Dev Neurosci, 2008. 26(1): p. 133-40.

475. Tomasik, T., et al., *[Intracranial hemorrhage in term newborn].* Przegl Lek, 2005. 62(11): p. 1227-35.

476. Aksoy, U., *Prenatal color Doppler sonographic evaluation of nuchal encirclement by the umbilical cord.* J Clin Ultrasound, 2003. 31(9): p. 473-7.

477. Clapp, J.F., 3rd, et al., *The natural history of antenatal nuchal cords.* Am J Obstet Gynecol, 2003. 189(2): p. 488-93.

478. Hanaoka, U., et al., *Comparison of three-dimensional, two-dimensional and color Doppler ultrasound in predicting the presence of a nuchal cord at birth.* Ultrasound Obstet Gynecol, 2002. 19(5): p. 471-4.

479. Nelson, K.B. and J.K. Grether, *Potentially asphyxiating conditions and spastic cerebral palsy in infants of normal birth weight.* Am J Obstet Gynecol, 1998. 179(2): p. 507-13.

480. Hansen, H.S. and B. Hillersborg, *Antepartum looping of the umbilical cord.* Acta Obstet Gynecol Scand, 1988. 67(5): p. 475-6.

481. Paul, R.H. and G. Krosnick, *Fetal heart rate in excessive cord encirclement.* Obstet Gynecol, 1966. 28(5): p. 646-9.

482. Sherer, D.M., et al., *Sonographic verification of a nuchal cord following a vibratory acoustic stimulation-induced severe variable fetal heart rate deceleration with expedient abdominal delivery.* Am J Perinatol, 1991. 8(5): p. 345-6.

483. Sherer, D.M., et al., *Prenatal sonographic diagnosis, assessment, and management of a fetus with a quadruple nuchal cord at 39 weeks' gestation.* Am J Perinatol, 1991. 8(6): p. 383-4.

484. Steinfeld, J.D., et al., *Prenatal detection and management of quadruple nuchal cord. A case report.* J Reprod Med, 1992. 37(12): p. 989-91.

485. Athanassiou, A., et al., *Is early antenatal diagnosis of a nuchal cord clinically useful?* Am J Obstet Gynecol, 2000. 182, SPO Abstract #360: p. 120.

486. Sanchez, A.G., L.S. Ortega, and J.G.P. Baron, *Valoracion de la compression del cordon en embarazos de riesgo normal por ultrasonografia y cardiotocografia.* Ginecol Obstet Mex, 1984. 52: p. 77-79.

487. Pilu, G., et al., *Sonographic demonstration of nuchal cord and abnormal umbilical artery waveform heralding fetal distress.* Ultrasound Obstet Gynecol, 1998. 12(2): p. 125-7.

488. Stembera, Z.K. and S. Horska, *The influence of coiling of the umbilical cord around the neck of the fetus on its gas metabolism and acid-base balance.* Biol Neonate, 1972. 20(3): p. 214-25.

489. Hankins, G.D., et al., *Nuchal cords and neonatal outcome.* Obstet Gynecol, 1987. 70(5): p. 687-91.

490. Roemer, V.M. and S. Kortum-Roemer, *THe impact of cord-entaglement on neonatal acid-base balance: observations and conclusions.* Z Geburtshilfe Perinatol, 1993. 197: p. 20-26.

491. Graczyk, S. and U. Kowalska-Koprek, *[Effect of umbilical cord compression on acid-base parameters in blood from the umbilical artery in neonates].* Ginekol Pol, 1994. 65(5): p. 227-9.

492. Jauniaux, E., et al., *Perinatal features of pregnancies complicated by nuchal cord.* Am J Perinatol, 1995. 12(4): p. 255-8.

493. Williams, J., G.H. Katzman, and S.S. Kripke, *Neck compression by nuchal cord.* Am J Obstet Gynecol, 1981. 140(3): p. 345-6.

494. Grimm, T.W. and T.A. Cable, *Nuchal cord: an unusual manifestation.* J Am Board Fam Pract, 1988. 1(3): p. 218-9.

495. Airas, U. and S. Heinonen, *Clinical significance of true umbilical knots: a population-based analysis.* Am J Perinatol, 2002. 19(3): p. 127-32.

496. Baz, E., et al., *Abnormal ductus venosus blood flow: a clue to umbilical cord complication.* Ultrasound Obstet Gynecol, 1999. 13(3): p. 204-6.

497. Qian, Z.L., *[Detection of umbilical coils around the fetal neck by Doppler's ultrasound technic (report of 112 cases) (author's transl)].* Zhonghua Fu Chan Ke Za Zhi, 1982. 17(1): p. 31.

498. Plasencia, W., *Nuchal Cord influence on ductous venosous assessment at 11-13+wks of gestation.* Ultrsound Obstet Gynecol, 2010(Jan 26).

499. Ghosh, G.S. and S. Gudmundsson, *Nuchal cord in post-term pregnancy - relationship to suspected intrapartum fetal distress indicating operative intervention.* J Perinat Med, 2008. 36(2): p. 142-4.

500. Corona-Rivera, J.R., et al., *Umbilical cord disruption sequence caused by long cord in two unrelated infants with amyoplasia.* Fetal Pediatr Pathol, 2009. 28(3): p. 101-8.

501. Wang, C., *Fetal asphyxia caused by umbilical cord anomalies.* Chinese J Obstet Gynecol, 1958. 6: p. 344-48.

502. Grishchenko, V.I. and G.S. Efimova, *[Current possibilities of diagnosis of twisting of the umbilical cord around the fetus' body].* Akush Ginekol (Mosk), 1984(10): p. 75-9.

503. Zhao, S., H. Dai, and D. Shao, *[Predictive value of combined application of umbilical artery color Doppler velocimetry,*

nonstress testing and ultrasonography in monitoring umbilical cord entanglement]. Zhonghua Yi Xue Za Zhi, 2001. 81(8): p. 468-71.

504. Hershkovitz, R., et al., *Risk factors associated with true knots of the umbilical cord.* Eur J Obstet Gynecol Reprod Biol, 2001. 98(1): p. 36-9.

505. Omari, A.A. and D. Cameron, *Getting knotted: umbilical knots in a monochorionic monoamniotic twin pregnancy.* Arch Dis Child Fetal Neonatal Ed, 2005. 90(1): p. F24.

506. Barigye, O., et al., *High risk of unexpected late fetal death in monochorionic twins despite intensive ultrasound surveillance: a cohort study.* PLoS Med, 2005. 2(6): p. e172.

507. Pijnenborg, J.M. and S.G. Oei, *The monoamniotic twin: a riskful event.* Eur J Obstet Gynecol Reprod Biol, 1999. 86(1): p. 51-3.

508. Deutsch, A.B., et al., *Ultrasound to identify cord knotting in monoamniotic monochorionic twins.* Twin Res Hum Genet, 2007. 10(1): p. 216-8.

509. Sornes, T., *Umbilical cord knots.* Acta Obstet Gynecol Scand, 2000. 79(3): p. 157-9.

510. Joura, A.E., H. Zeisler, and M.O. Sator, *Epidemiologie und klinische Wertigkeit von echten Nabelschnurknoten.* Wein Klin Wochenschr, 1998. 110: p. 232-35.

511. Maher, J.T. and J.A. Conti, *A comparison of umbilical cord blood gas values between newborns with and without true knots.* Obstet Gynecol, 1996. 88(5): p. 863-6.

512. Sopracordevole, F. and M.G. Perissinotto, *Il nodo vero di funicolo: implicazioni cliniche.* Minerva Ginecol, 1991. 43: p. 109-13.

513. Blickstein, I., Z. Shoham-Schwartz, and M. Lancet, *Predisposing factors in the formation of true knots of the umbilical cord--analysis of morphometric and perinatal data.* Int J Gynaecol Obstet, 1987. 25(5): p. 395-8.

514. Roberts, R.N., *Combined simple and complex cord knots.* Eur J Obstet Gynecol Reprod Biol, 1995. 62(1): p. 131-3.

515. Robins, J.B., *A complex true knot of the umbilical cord.* Br J Clin Pract, 1995. 49(3): p. 164-5.

516. Jakabi, P., et al., *Systolic notch in umbilical artery flow waveforms associated with a tight knot of the cord.* J Matern-Fetal Invest, 1994. 4: p. 119-121.

517. Barreca, P. and S. Damiani, *A rare case of ante partum fetal death due to funicular pathology.* Acta Eur Fertil, 1977. 8(3): p. 257-64.

518. Iglesias, J., et al., *[Meconium in the amnioscopy and true knot of the umbilical cord. Critical analysis of 2 cases].* Rev Chil Obstet Ginecol, 1971. 36(4): p. 193-5.

519. Frumkin, A., *Herpes gestationis, umbilical cord knot, and fetal death.* J Am Acad Dermatol, 1989. 21(4 Pt 1): p. 812-3.

520. Collins, J.H., *Two cases of multiple umbilical cord abnormalities resulting in stillbirth: prenatal observation with ultrasonography and fetal heart rates.* Am J Obstet Gynecol, 1993. 168(1 Pt 1): p. 125-8.

521. Collins, J.C., R.J. Muller, and C.L. Collins, *Prenatal observation of umbilical cord abnormalities: a triple knot and torsion of the umbilical cord.* Am J Obstet Gynecol, 1993. 169(1): p. 102-4.

522. Abitol, M.M., et al., *Diagnosis of umbilical cord compression by Doppler velocimetry.* J Mater Fetal Invest, 1994. 12: p. 257-61.

523. Hales, E.D. and L.S. Westney, *Sonography of occult cord prolapse.* J Clin Ultrasound, 1984. 12(5): p. 283-5.

524. Sakamoto, H., et al., *Clinical application of the perineal scan: prepartum screening for cord presentation.* Am J Obstet Gynecol, 1986. 155(5): p. 1041-3.

525. Raga, F., et al., *Color flow Doppler: a useful instrument in the diagnosis of funic presentation.* J Natl Med Assoc, 1996. 88(2): p. 94-6.

526. Murphy, D.J. and I.Z. MacKenzie, *The mortality and morbidity associated with umbilical cord prolapse.* Br J Obstet Gynaecol, 1995. 102(10): p. 826-30.

527. Prabulos, A.M. and E.H. Philipson, *Umbilical cord prolapse. Is the time from diagnosis to delivery critical?* J Reprod Med, 1998. 43(2): p. 129-32.

528. Pelosi, M.A., *Antepartum ultrasonic diagnosis of cord presentation.* Am J Obstet Gynecol, 1990. 162(2): p. 599-601.

529. Barrett, J.M., *Funic reduction for the management of umbilical cord prolapse.* Am J Obstet Gynecol, 1991. 165(3): p. 654-7.

530. Jones, G., S. Grenier, and A. Gruslin, *Sonographic diagnosis of funic presentation: implications for delivery.* BJOG, 2000. 107(8): p. 1055-7.

531. Gimovsky, M.L. and C. Boyd, *Funic presentation as a complication of external cephalic version. A case report.* J Reprod Med, 1999. 44(10): p. 897-8.

532. Freistadt, H., *Fetal heart rate monitoring casebook. Nonreassuring fetal heart rate, attempted instrumental delivery, forceps rotation, cord prolapse during rotation maneuver, and rescue by extreme emergency abdominal delivery.* J Perinatol, 2001. 21(1): p. 76-8.

533. Wu, P., L. Song, and X.Y. Tang, *[Clinical observation of the relationship between puerperant posture and occult prolapse of cord].* Zhonghua Hu Li Za Zhi, 1996. 31(6): p. 335-6.

534. Oyelese, Y., et al., *Persistent funic presentation resulting from marginal cord insertion into a low-lying placenta.* Ultrasound Obstet Gynecol, 2004. 24(6): p. 692-3.

535. Palsdottir, K., et al., *[Birth asphyxia and hypoxic ischemic encephalopathy, incidence and obstetric risk factors].* Laeknabladid, 2007. 93(9): p. 595-601.

536. Ito, T., et al., *Clinical features of and cardiotocographic findings for premature infants with antenatal periventricular leukomalacia.* Early Hum Dev, 1997. 47(2): p. 195-201.

537. Williams, M.C., *Nuchal cords and cord knots predispose to altered fetal growth.* Am J Obstet Gynecol, 2000. 182, SPO Abstracts #188: p. 73.

538. Sornes, T., *Umbilical cord encirclements and fetal growth restriction.* Obstet Gynecol, 1995. 86(5): p. 725-8.

539. Osak, R., et al., *Nuchal cord evident at birth impacts on fetal size relative to that of the placenta.* Early Hum Dev, 1997. 49(3): p. 193-202.

540. Falkowski, A., et al., *Apoptosis in the preterm and near term ovine fetal brain and the effect of intermittent umbilical cord occlusion.* Brain Res Dev Brain Res, 2002. 136(2): p. 165-73.

541. Romero Gutierrez, G., et al., *[Color Doppler flowmetry values in fetuses with nuchal cord encirclement]*. Ginecol Obstet Mex, 2000. 68: p. 401-7.

542. Bruce, S., et al., *Umbilical cord complications as a cause of perinatal morbidity and mortality.* J Perinat Med, 1978. 6(2): p. 89-94.

543. Li, S.R. and L.C. Ying, *Dystocia by the umbilical cord.* Chinese J Obstet Gynecol, 1956. 4: p. 45-50.

544. Zhang, J. and M.A. Klebanoff, *Low blood pressure during pregnancy and poor perinatal outcomes: an obstetric paradox.* Am J Epidemiol, 2001. 153(7): p. 642-6.

545. Eifinger, F., et al., *Neonatal Testicular Infarction-Possibly due to Compression of the Umbilical Cord?* Urology, 2009.

546. Khurana, A., P.C. Huettner, and F.S. Cole, *Umbilical cord ulceration as a cause of hypoxic-ischemic encephalopathy: report of a case and review of the literature.* J Perinatol, 1995. 15(5): p. 423-5.

547. Coulter, J.B.S., J.M. Scott, and M.M. Jordan, *Edema of the cord and respiratory distress in the newborn.* Br J Obstet and Gynaecol, 1975. 82: p. 453-59.

548. Matsuda, T., et al., *Necrotizing funisitis: clinical significance and association with chronic lung disease in premature infants.* Am J Obstet Gynecol, 1997. 177(6): p. 1402-7.

549. Lira, D.O., et al., *Stenosis of the umbilical cord and nonimmunologic hydrops fetalis.* Ginecol Obstet Mex, 1988. 56: p. 277-80.

550. Collins, J.H., *Prenatal observation of umbilical cord torsion with subsequent premature labor and delivery of a 31-week*

infant with mild nonimmune hydrops. Am J Obstet Gynecol, 1995. 172(3): p. 1048-9.

551. Burgess, A.M. and G.M. Hutchins, *Inflammation of the lungs, umbilical cord and placenta associated with meconium passage in utero. Review of 123 autopsied cases.* Pathol Res Pract, 1996. 192(11): p. 1121-8.

552. Lazda, E.J., W.H. Batchelor, and P.M. Cox, *Immunohistochemical detection of myocardial necrosis in stillbirth and neonatal death.* Pediatr Dev Pathol, 2000. 3(1): p. 40-7.

553. Tsivyan, P.B. and A.D. Vasenina, *Left ventricular systolic and diastolic function in term neonates after mild perinatal asphyxia.* Eur J Obstet Gynecol Reprod Biol, 1991. 40(2): p. 105-10.

554. Ikeda, T., et al., *Histologic and biochemical study of the brain, heart, kidney, and liver in asphyxia caused by occlusion of the umbilical cord in near-term fetal lambs.* Am J Obstet Gynecol, 2000. 182(2): p. 449-57.

555. Thureen, P.J., et al., *Fatal meconium aspiration in spite of appropriate perinatal airway management: pulmonary and placental evidence of prenatal disease.* Am J Obstet Gynecol, 1997. 176(5): p. 967-75.

556. Shaikh, S., et al., *Diffuse unilateral hemorrhagic retinopathy associated with accidental perinatal strangulation. A clinicopathologic report.* Retina, 2001. 21(3): p. 252-5.

557. Kosmarskaya, E.N., B.E. G., and T.P. Zhukova, *The influence of asphyxia on the function of the developing vestibulo-oculomotor system.* Vestnik Otorinolaringologii, 1968. 30: p. 31-37.

558. Low, J.A., *Intrapartum fetal asphyxia: definition, diagnosis, and classification.* Am J Obstet Gynecol, 1997. 176(5): p. 957-9.

559. van den Berg, P.P., et al., *Neonatal complications in newborns with an umbilical artery pH < 7.00.* Am J Obstet Gynecol, 1996. 175(5): p. 1152-7.

560. Hofmeyr, G.J., et al., *Periventricular/intraventricular haemorrhage and umbilical cord clamping. Findings and hypothesis.* S Afr Med J, 1988. 73(2): p. 104-6.

561. Varangot, J., et al., *La souffrance cerbrale du nouveau-ne a terme, causes et devenir.* Nouv Presse Med, 1975. 4: p. 1257-62.

562. Clapp, J.F., 3rd, B. Lopez, and S. Simonean, *Nuchal cord and neurodevelopmental performance at 1 year.* J Soc Gynecol Investig, 1999. 6(5): p. 268-72.

563. Gunther-Genta, F., P. Bovet, and P. Hohlfeld, *Obstetrical complications and schizophrenia: a case-control study.* BMJ, 1994. 164: p. 165-170.

564. Collins, J.H. and C.L. Collins, *Umbilical cord compression, persistent pulmonary hypertension, and placental villous hypervascularity.* Am J Obstet Gynecol, 1997. 177(5): p. 1276-7.

565. Akinbi, H., et al., *Gastrointestinal and renal blood flow velocity profile in neonates with birth asphyxia.* J Pediatr, 1994. 125(4): p. 625-7.

566. Redline, R.W., *Inflammatory responses in the placenta and umbilical cord.* Semin Fetal Neonatal Med, 2006. 11(5): p. 296-301.

567. Redline, R.W., *Disorders of placental circulation and the fetal brain.* Clin Perinatol, 2009. 36(3): p. 549-59.

568. Benirschke, K., *Timing Fetal Injury: The Role of the Placenta.* OBG Management, 2000. March: p. 72-87.

569. Magee, J.F., *Investigation of stillbirth.* Pediatr Dev Pathol, 2001. 4(1): p. 1-22.

570. Redline, R.W., *Elevated circulating fetal nucleated red blood cells and placental pathology in term infants who develop cerebral palsy.* Hum Pathol, 2008. 39(9): p. 1378-84.

571. Naeye, R.L. and H.M. Lin, *Determination of the timing of fetal brain damage from hypoxemia-ischemia.* Am J Obstet Gynecol, 2001. 184(2): p. 217-24.

572. Koen, S., et al., *Prevalence of organ system injury in acute birth asphyxia.* Am J Obstet Gynecol, 2001. 184: p. SPO Abstract #439, S133.

573. Phelan, J.P., et al., *Intrapartum fetal asphyxia: could the brain be injured first?* Am J Obstet Gynecol, 1995. 172, SPO Abstract #379: p. 364.

574. Vintzileos, A.M. and R.A. Knuppel, *Multiple parameter biophysical testing in the prediction of fetal acid-base status.* Clin Perinatol, 1994. 21(4): p. 823-48.

575. Grafe, M.R., *The correlation of prenatal brain damage with placental pathology.* J Neuropathol Exp Neurol, 1994. 53(4): p. 407-15.

576. Walsh, F.B. and R. Lindenberg, *Hypoxia in infants and children: a clinical-pathological study concerning the primary visual pathways.* Bull Johns Hopkins Hosp, 1961. 108: p. 100-45.

577. Daniel, S.S., et al., *Renal response of the lamb fetus to partial occlusion of the umbilical cord.* J Pediatr, 1975. 87(5): p. 788-94.

578. Daniel, S.S., et al., *Renal response of fetal lamb to complete occlusion of umbilical cord.* Am J Obstet Gynecol, 1978. 131(5): p. 514-9.

579. Ogundipe, O.A., et al., *Fetal endocrine and renal responses to in utero ventilation and umbilical cord occlusion.* Am J Obstet Gynecol, 1993. 169(6): p. 1479-86.

580. Gunn, A.J., et al., *Delayed hypotension and subendocardial injury after repeated umbilical cord occlusion in near-term fetal lambs.* Am J Obstet Gynecol, 2000. 183(6): p. 1564-72.

581. Mallard, E.C., et al., *Repeated episodes of umbilical cord occlusion in fetal sheep lead to preferential damage to the striatum and sensitize the heart to further insults.* Pediatr Res, 1995. 37(6): p. 707-13.

582. Terzidou, V. and P. Bennett, *Maternal risk factors for fetal and neonatal brain damage.* Biol Neonate, 2001. 79(3-4): p. 157-62.

583. Marumo, G., et al., *Generation of periventricular leukomalacia by repeated umbilical cord occlusion in near-term fetal sheep and its possible pathogenetical mechanisms.* Biol Neonate, 2001. 79(1): p. 39-45.

584. Clapp, J.F., et al., *Brain damage after intermittent partial cord occlusion in the chronically instrumented fetal lamb.* Am J Obstet Gynecol, 1988. 159(2): p. 504-9.

585. Keunen, H., et al., *Absence of neuronal damage after umbilical cord occlusion of 10, 15, and 20 minutes in midgestation fetal sheep.* Am J Obstet Gynecol, 1997. 176(3): p. 515-20.

586. Keunen, H., et al., *Effect of repetitive umbilical cord occlusions on neuronal brain activity measured by the cerebral function analyzing monitor and histologic outcome in immature fetal sheep.* J Soc Gynecol Investig, 2000. 7(4): p. 218-23.

587. De Haan, H.H., et al., *Brief repeated umbilical cord occlusions cause sustained cytotoxic cerebral edema and focal infarcts in near-term fetal lambs.* Pediatr Res, 1997. 41(1): p. 96-104.

588. Soifer, S.J., et al., *Umbilical cord compression produces pulmonary hypertension in newborn lambs: a model to study the pathophysiology of persistent pulmonary hypertension in the newborn.* J Dev Physiol, 1987. 9(3): p. 239-52.

589. Bennet, L., et al., *Pathophysiology of Asphyxia Ch 5.* Fetal and Neonatal Neurology and Neurosurgery (ed 3), ed. M. Levene, et al. 2001: 407-426, London, England: Harcourt Health Sciences

590. Anagnostakis, D., et al., *Umbilical cord entanglement: a cause of neonatal pulmonary haemorrhage?* Helv Paediatr Acta, 1974. 29(2): p. 167-71.

591. Todd, A.L., et al., *Antenatal tests of fetal welfare and development at age 2 years.* Am J Obstet Gynecol, 1992. 167(1): p. 66-71.

592. Avignon, J., R.R. Lorenz, and J.T. Shepherd, *Response of human umbilical artery to changes in transmural pressure.* Am J Physiol, 1965. 209(1): p. 1-9.

593. Dawes, G.S., *Fetal and Neonatal Physiology: a comparative study of the changes at birth.* 1968; 160-161, Chicago, IL: Year Book Medical Publishers.

594. Muppala H, B.-R.A., Martindale E, *Abnormally Long Umbilical Cord with Marked Spiraling and True Knots: A Case Report.* The Internet Journal of Gynecology and Obstetrics, 2007. 7(2): p. 1.

595. de Vries, J.I. and B.F. Fong, *Changes in fetal motility as a result of congenital disorders: an overview.* Ultrasound Obstet Gynecol, 2007. 29(5): p. 590-9.

596. de Vries, J.I. and B.F. Fong, *Normal fetal motility: an overview.* Ultrasound Obstet Gynecol, 2006. 27(6): p. 701-11.

597. van Kan, C.M., et al., *Ontogeny of fetal movements in the guinea pig.* Physiol Behav, 2009. 98(3): p. 338-44.

598. Kurjak, A., et al., *The potential of four-dimensional (4D) ultrasonography in the assessment of fetal awareness.* J Perinat Med, 2005. 33(1): p. 46-53.

599. Smotherman, W.P. and S.R. Robinson, *Response of the rat fetus to acute umbilical cord occlusion: an ontogenetic adaptation?* Physiol Behav, 1988. 44(1): p. 131-5.

600. Harman, C.R., *Invasive Techniques in the Management of Alloimmune Anemia.* Invasive Fetal Testing and Treatment, ed. C.R. Harman. 1995. p 109-191 (Fig 6-34A), Cambridge, MA: Blackwell Scientific Publishers.

601. Rayburn, W.F., P.R. Rayburn, and L.L. Gabel, *Excessive fetal activity: another worrisome sign?* South Med J, 1983. 76(2): p. 163-5.

602. Patrick, J., et al., *Patterns of gross fetal body movements over 24-hour observation intervals during the last 10 weeks of pregnancy.* Am J Obstet Gynecol, 1982. 142(4): p. 363-71.

603. Hems, D.A., *Palpable regular jerking movements of the human fetus: a possible respiratory sign of fetal distress.* Biol Neonate, 1973. 23(3): p. 223-30.

604. Collins, J., *Fetal hiccups and the umbilical ring.* Am J Obstet Gynecol, 1991. 165(4 Pt 1): p. 1161.

605. Woudstra, B.R., et al., *Nuchal muscle activity at different levels of hypoxemia in fetal sheep.* Am J Obstet Gynecol, 1990. 162(2): p. 559-64.

606. Zheng, Y.T., M.B. Sampson, and R. Soper, *The Significance of Umbilical Vein Doppler Changes during Fetal Hiccups.* J Matern Fetal Investig, 1998. 8(2): p. 89-91.

607. Popescu, E.A., et al., *Magnetographic assessment of fetal hiccups and their effect on fetal heart rhythm.* Physiol Meas, 2007. 28(6): p. 665-76.

608. Sadovsky, E., et al., *Decreased fetal movements associated with umbilical cord complications.* Isr J Med Sci, 1977. 13(3): p. 295-8.

609. Leader, L.R., P. Baillie, and D.J. Van Schalkwyk, *Fetal movements and fetal outcome: a prospective study.* Obstet Gynecol, 1981. 57(4): p. 431-6.

610. Patrick, J., *Fetal Breathing and body Movements.* Maternal Fetal Medicine Principles and Practice, ed. R.K. Creasy and R. Resnik. 1984. 239-257, Philadelphia, PA: W B Saunders.

611. Efkarpidis, S., et al., *Case-control study of factors associated with intrauterine fetal deaths.* MedGenMed, 2004. 6(2): p. 53.

612. Minors, D.S. and J.M. Waterhouse, *The effect of maternal posture, meals and time of day on fetal movements.* Br J Obstet Gynaecol, 1979. 86(9): p. 717-23.

613. Ehrstrom, C., *Circadian rhythm of fetal movements.* Acta Obstet Gynecol Scand, 1984. 63(6): p. 539-41.

614. Romanini, C. and G. Rizzo, *Fetal behaviour in normal and compromised fetuses. An overview.* Early Hum Dev, 1995. 43(2): p. 117-31.

615. Flenady, V., et al., *Detection and management of decreased fetal movements in Australia and New Zealand: a survey of obstetric practice.* Aust N Z J Obstet Gynaecol, 2009. 49(4): p. 358-63.

616. Tveit, J.V., et al., *Reduction of late stillbirth with the introduction of fetal movement information and guidelines - a clinical quality improvement.* BMC Pregnancy Childbirth, 2009. 9: p. 32.

617. Froen, J.F., et al., *Management of decreased fetal movements.* Semin Perinatol, 2008. 32(4): p. 307-11.

618. Robson, S.J. and L.R. Leader, *Management of subsequent pregnancy after an unexplained stillbirth.* J Perinatol, 2009.

619. Haws, R.A., et al., *Reducing stillbirths: screening and monitoring during pregnancy and labour.* BMC Pregnancy Childbirth, 2009. 9 Suppl 1: p. S5.

620. Olesen, A.G. and J.A. Svare, *Decreased fetal movements: background, assessment, and clinical management.* Acta Obstet Gynecol Scand, 2004. 83(9): p. 818-26.

621. Vintzileos, A.M., et al., *Relationship between fetal biophysical activities and umbilical cord blood gas values.* Am J Obstet Gynecol, 1991. 165(3): p. 707-13.

622. Poets, C.F., et al., *Gasping and other cardiorespiratory patterns during sudden infant deaths.* Pediatr Res, 1999. 45(3): p. 350-4.

623. Gozal, D. and J.E. Torres, *Brainstem nitric oxide tissue levels correlate with anoxia-induced gasping activity in the developing rat.* Biol Neonate, 2001. 79(2): p. 122-30.

624. Yan, E.B., et al., *Changes in cerebral blood flow, cerebral metabolites, and breathing movements in the sheep fetus following asphyxia produced by occlusion of the umbilical cord.* Am J Physiol Regul Integr Comp Physiol, 2009. 297(1): p. R60-9.

625. Bakker, P.C. and H.P. van Geijn, *Uterine activity: implications for the condition of the fetus.* J Perinat Med, 2008. 36(1): p. 30-7.

626. Ducros, L., et al., *Increasing maternal blood pressure with ephedrine increases uterine artery blood flow velocity during uterine contraction.* Anesthesiology, 2002. 96(3): p. 612-6.

627. Bakker, P.C., S. Van Rijswijk, and H.P. van Geijn, *Uterine activity monitoring during labor.* J Perinat Med, 2007. 35(6): p. 468-77.

628. Yoon, B.H., et al., *Tetanic uterine contraction may be a cause of persistent fetal bradycardia after fetal blood sampling by ultrasound-guided cordocentesis.* Asia Oceania J Obstet Gynaecol, 1992. 18(3): p. 207-9.

629. Bakker, P.C., et al., *Elevated uterine activity increases the risk of fetal acidosis at birth.* Am J Obstet Gynecol, 2007. 196(4): p. 313 e1-6.

630. Watson, C.S., et al., *Effect of intermittent umbilical cord occlusion on fetal respiratory activity and brain adenosine in late-gestation sheep.* Reprod Fertil Dev, 2002. 14(1-2): p. 35-42.

631. Cabaniss, M.L., *Fetal monitoring Interpretation.* 1992, Philadelphia, PA: J B Lippincott.

632. Ingemarsson, I., E. Ingemarsson, and J.A.D. Spencer, *Fetal heart rate monitoring, a practical guide.* 1993, N.Y., N.Y.: Oxford University Press.

633. Hanson, M.A., J.A.D. Spencer, and C.H. Rodeck, *Neonatal Physiology and Clinical Applications. Vol I The Circulation.* 1993, N.Y., N.Y.: Cambridge University Press.

634. Thornburn, G.D. and R. Harding, *Textbook of Fetal Physiology.* 1994, N.Y., N.Y.: Oxford Medical Press.

635. Ball, R.H. and J.T. Parer, *The physiologic mechanisms of variable decelerations.* Am J Obstet Gynecol, 1992. 166(6 Pt 1): p. 1683-8; discussion 1688-9.

636. Saito, J., et al., *Alteration of FHR pattern associated with progressively advanced fetal acidemia caused by cord compression.* Nippon Sanka Fujinka Gakkai Zasshi, 1988. 40(6): p. 775-80.

637. Lee, C.Y., P.C. Di Loreto, and J.M. O'Lane, *A study of fetal heart rate acceleration patterns.* Obstet Gynecol, 1975. 45(2): p. 142-6.

638. Krebs, H.B., R.E. Petres, and L.J. Dunn, *Intrapartum fetal heart rate monitoring. VIII. Atypical variable decelerations.* Am J Obstet Gynecol, 1983. 145(3): p. 297-305.

639. Itskovitz, J., E.F. LaGamma, and A.M. Rudolph, *Heart rate and blood pressure responses to umbilical cord compression in fetal lambs with special reference to the mechanism of variable deceleration.* Am J Obstet Gynecol, 1983. 147(4): p. 451-7.

640. Westgate, J.A., L. Bennet, and A.J. Gunn, *Fetal heart rate variability changes during brief repeated umbilical cord occlusion in near term fetal sheep.* Br J Obstet Gynaecol, 1999. 106(7): p. 664-71.

641. Simmons, J.N., P. Rufleth, and P.E. Lewis, *Identification of nuchal cords during nonstress testing.* J Reprod Med, 1985. 30(2): p. 97-100.

642. Welt, S.I., *The fetal heart rate W-sign.* Obstet Gynecol, 1984. 63(3): p. 405-8.

643. Brubaker, K. and T.J. Garite, *The lambda fetal heart rate pattern: an assessment of its significance in the intrapartum period.* Obstet Gynecol, 1988. 72(6): p. 881-5.

644. Goodlin, R.C. and E.W. Lowe, *A functional umbilical cord occlusion heart rate pattern. The significance of overshoot.* Obstet Gynecol, 1974. 43(1): p. 22-30.

645. Odendaal, H.J. and J.V. Van der Merwe, *Abrupt fall in the fetal heart rate during labour.* S Afr Med J, 1976. 50(49): p. 1960-2.

646. Selbing, A., *Umbilical cord compression diagnosed by means of ultrasound.* Acta Obstet Gynecol Scand, 1988. 67(6): p. 565-7.

647. Chen, S.Z., et al., *Fetal supraventricular tachycardia associated with a true knot of umbilical cord.* Asia Oceania J Obstet Gynaecol, 1987. 13(1): p. 69-74.

648. Gabbe, S.G., et al., *Umbilical cord compression associated with amniotomy: laboratory observations.* Am J Obstet Gynecol, 1976. 126(3): p. 353-5.

649. Miyazaki, F.S. and F. Nevarez, *Saline amnioinfusion for relief of repetitive variable decelerations: a prospective randomized study.* Am J Obstet Gynecol, 1985. 153(3): p. 301-6.

650. Hofmeyr, G.J., *Amnioinfusion for umbilical cord compression in labour.* Cochrane Database Syst Rev, 2000. 2: p. CD0000013.

651. Brotanek, V. and J.S. Lopez, *An unusual cause and treatment of decelerations in fetal heart rate.* Int J Gynaecol Obstet, 1991. 34(3): p. 271-5.

652. Collins, J.H., *Fetal grasping of the umbilical cord with simultaneous fetal heart rate monitoring.* Am J Obstet Gynecol, 1994. 170(6): p. 1836.

653. Heyl, W. and W. Rath, *[Intrapartum therapy-resistant fetal bradycardia--color Doppler sonographic diagnosis of umbilical cord compression due to fetal grasping].* Z Geburtshilfe Neonatol, 1996. 200(1): p. 30-2.

654. Petrikovsky, B.M. and G.P. Kaplan, *Fetal grasping of the umbilical cord causing variable fetal heart rate decelerations.* J Clin Ultrasound, 1993. 21(9): p. 642-4.

655. *Electronic fetal heart rate monitoring: research guidelines for interpretation. National Institute of Child Health and Human Development Research Planning Workshop.* Am J Obstet Gynecol, 1997. 177(6): p. 1385-90.

656. Parer, J.T. and T. King, *Fetal heart rate monitoring: is it salvageable?* Am J Obstet Gynecol, 2000. 182(4): p. 982-7.

657. Collins, J.H., *Umbilical cord vulnerability.* Am J Obstet Gynecol, 2001. 184(4): p. 776.

658. Sisco, K.M., et al., *Is continuous monitoring the answer to incidentally observed fetal heart rate decelerations?* J Matern Fetal Neonatal Med, 2009. 22(5): p. 405-9.

659. Mohide, P. and M.J.N.C. Keirse, *Methods of Biophysical Assessment in Effective Care in Pregnancy and Childbirth,*

ed. I. Chalmers, M. Enkin, and M.J.N.C. Keirse. 1989; 1:480, Oxford, England: Oxford University Press.

660. van Heeswijk, M., J.G. Nijhuis, and H.M. Hollanders, *Fetal heart rate in early pregnancy.* Early Hum Dev, 1990. 22(3): p. 151-6.

661. Pillai, M. and D. James, *The development of fetal heart rate patterns during normal pregnancy.* Obstet Gynecol, 1990. 76(5 Pt 1): p. 812-6.

662. Ursem, N.T., et al., *An estimate of fetal autonomic state by spectral analysis of human umbilical artery flow velocity waveforms.* Cardiovasc Res, 1998. 37(3): p. 601-5.

663. Ursem, N.T., et al., *Heart rate and flow velocity variability as determined from umbilical Doppler velocimetry at 10-20 weeks of gestation.* Clin Sci (Lond), 1998. 95(5): p. 539-45.

664. Hasegawa, J., et al., *Atypical variable deceleration in the first stage of labor is a characteristic fetal heart-rate pattern for velamentous cord insertion and hypercoiled cord.* J Obstet Gynaecol Res, 2009. 35(1): p. 35-9.

665. Odendaal, H.J., *Die Invloed van Naelstringbeklemming op die Fetale Hartfrekwensie.* S A Med J Obstet Gynecol, 1976. 62: p. 1966-68.

666. Ransom, S.B., et al., *Reduced medicolegal risk by compliance with obstetric clinical pathways: a case-control study.* Obstet Gynecol, 2003. 101(4): p. 751-5.

667. Phelan, J.P. and P.E. Lewis, Jr., *Fetal heart rate decelerations during a nonstress test.* Obstet Gynecol, 1981. 57(2): p. 228-32.

668. Bruce, S.L., R.H. Petrie, and J. Davison, *Prediction of abnormal umbilical cord position and intrapartum cord*

problems from the nonstress test. Diagn Gynecol Obstet, 1980. 2(1): p. 47-9.

669. O'Leary, J.A., G.C. Andrinopoulos, and P.C. Giordano, *Variable decelerations and the nonstress test: an indication of cord compromise.* Am J Obstet Gynecol, 1980. 137(6): p. 704-6.

670. Troeger, C., V. Briese, and H. Muller, *[Validity of cardiotocography in the detection of umbilical cord complications].* Zentralbl Gynakol, 1999. 121(5): p. 233-8.

671. Shi, G. and S.W. Wang, *[Fetal heart rate monitoring in the prenatal diagnosis of cord position abnormalities].* Zhonghua Fu Chan Ke Za Zhi, 1993. 28(11): p. 662-4, 701.

672. Logvinenko, A.V., et al., *[Possibilities of prenatal diagnosis of umbilical pathology by ultrasonic examination and cardiotocography].* Akush Ginekol (Mosk), 1988(1): p. 26-7.

673. Goldkrand, J.W. and J.P. Speichinger, *"Mixed cord compression," fetal heart rate pattern, and its relation to abnormal cord position.* Am J Obstet Gynecol, 1975. 122(2): p. 144-50.

674. Doig, J.R., et al., *Fetal cardiac electromechanical intervals during labour and effects of hypoxia and cord compression.* Br J Obstet Gynaecol, 1982. 89(2): p. 145-8.

675. Yeh, M.N., et al., *Myocardial conduction defects in association with compression of the umbilical cord. Experimental observations on fetal baboons.* Am J Obstet Gynecol, 1975. 121(7): p. 951-7.

676. Westgate, J.A., et al., *Do fetal electrocardiogram PR-RR changes reflect progressive asphyxia after repeated umbilical cord occlusion in fetal sheep?* Pediatr Res, 1998. 44(3): p. 297-303.

677. Keunen, H., et al., *The PR interval-fetal heart rate relationship during repetitive umbilical cord occlusions in immature fetal sheep.* Eur J Obstet Gynecol Reprod Biol, 2000. 89(1): p. 69-74.

678. Evertson, L.R., R.J. Gauthier, and J.V. Collea, *Fetal demise following negative contraction stress tests.* Obstet Gynecol, 1978. 51(6): p. 671-3.

679. Charonis, N.G., *Cord involvement bradycardia.* Intl J Obstet Gynecol, 1973. 11: p. 5-10.

680. Boehm, F.H., *Prolonged end stage fetal heart rate deceleration.* Obstet Gynecol, 1975. 45(5): p. 579-82.

681. Shaxted, E.J. and H.M. Jenkins, *Fetal death immediately following normal antenatal fetal heart rate pattern. Case report.* Br J Obstet Gynaecol, 1981. 88(7): p. 747-8.

682. Shuping, Z.H.A.O., et al. *Predictive value of combined application of umbilical artery color Doppler velocimetry, nonstress testing and ultrasonography in monitoring umbilical entanglement.* Natl Med J China, 2001. 81: p. 468-70.

683. Johnson, N. and V.A. Johnson, *Continuous fetal monitoring with a pulse oximeter: a case of cord compression.* Am J Obstet Gynecol, 1989. 161(5): p. 1295-6.

684. Bergmans, M.G., et al., *Transcutaneous and arterial carbon dioxide tension during intermittent umbilical cord occlusion in fetal sheep.* Gynecol Obstet Invest, 1997. 43(3): p. 150-4.

685. Habek, D., et al., *Fetal grasping of the umbilical cord and perinatal outcome.* Arch Gynecol Obstet, 2003. 268(4): p. 274-7.

686. Jakobovits, A., *[Grasping reflex activity in utero is one element of fetal behavior (Grasping activity is a part of fetal ethology)]*. Orv Hetil, 2007. 148(35): p. 1673-5.

687. Jakobovits, A.A., *Grasping activity in utero: a significant indicator of fetal behavior (The role of the grasping reflex in fetal ethology)*. J Perinat Med, 2009.

688. Sherer, D.M., *Fetal grasping at 16 weeks' gestation*. J Ultrasound Med, 1993. 12(6): p. 316.

689. Petrikovsky, B., *Fetal grasping of the umbilical cord*. Am J Obstet Gynecol, 1995. 172(3): p. 1071.

690. Habek, D., et al., *3D-ultrasound detection of fetal grasping of the umbilical cord and fetal outcome*. Fetal Diagn Ther, 2006. 21(4): p. 332-3.

691. Weber, M.A., et al., *Third trimester intrauterine fetal death caused by arterial aneurysm of the umbilical cord*. Pediatr Dev Pathol, 2007. 10(4): p. 305-8.

692. Barbati, A., et al., *Umbilical cord haematoma with altered fetal heart rate*. J Obstet Gynaecol, 2009. 29(2): p. 150-1.

693. LIU, B.N., *Pathologic Analysis of 76 Placentae in fetal distress*. Zhonghua Fu Chan Ke Za Zhi, 1991. 26(3): p. 144-8.

694. Amer-Wahlin, I., et al., *Fetal cerebral energy metabolism and electrocardiogram during experimental umbilical cord occlusion and resuscitation*. J Matern Fetal Neonatal Med, 2009: p. 1-9.

695. Richardson, B.S., et al., *Fetal cerebral, circulatory, and metabolic responses during heart rate decelerations with umbilical cord compression*. Am J Obstet Gynecol, 1996. 175(4 Pt 1): p. 929-36.

696. Lotgering, F.K., et al., *Ten-minute umbilical cord occlusion markedly reduces cerebral blood flow and heat production in fetal sheep.* Am J Obstet Gynecol, 2003. 189(1): p. 233-8.

697. Lu, G., et al., *Changes in the Tei index during acute fetal hypoxemia in the near-term ovine fetus after intermittent umbilical cord occlusion.* Ultrasound Obstet Gynecol, 2007.

698. Bennet, L. and A.J. Gunn, *The fetal heart rate response to hypoxia: insights from animal models.* Clin Perinatol, 2009. 36(3): p. 655-72.

699. Ikeda, T., et al., *Physiologic and histologic changes in near-term fetal lambs exposed to asphyxia by partial umbilical cord occlusion.* Am J Obstet Gynecol, 1998. 178(1 Pt 1): p. 24-32.

700. Ball, R.H., et al., *Regional blood flow and metabolism in ovine fetuses during severe cord occlusion.* Am J Obstet Gynecol, 1994. 171(6): p. 1549-55.

701. Kaneko, M., et al., *Cerebral blood flow and metabolism in relation to electrocortical activity with severe umbilical cord occlusion in the near-term ovine fetus.* Am J Obstet Gynecol, 2003. 188(4): p. 961-72.

702. Kawagoe, Y., et al., *Intermittent umbilical cord occlusion in the ovine fetus near term: effects on behavioral state activity.* Am J Obstet Gynecol, 1999. 181(6): p. 1520-9.

703. Bocking, A.D., *The relationship between heart rate and asphyxia in the animal fetus.* Clin Invest Med, 1993. 16(2): p. 166-75.

704. Nardo, L., et al., *The effect of repeated umbilical cord occlusions on pulmonary surfactant protein mRNA levels in the ovine fetus.* J Soc Gynecol Investig, 2005. 12(7): p. 510-7.

705. Reynolds, S.R.M., *The Umbilical Cord.* Scientific American, 1952. 187: p. 70-74.

706. Veth, A.F.L., *Modelling the Foetal Circulation: Simulation of the response to umbilical cord occlusion.* 1976, Utrecht, The Netherlands: Institute of Medical Physics TNO.

707. Constantino, M.L. and F. Miglietta, *Blood circulation in the fetal side of the human placenta: a mathematical model to investigate the effects induced by resistive pathologies.* J Mater Fetal Invest, 1996. 6: p. 199-206.

708. Hill, A.A., et al., *A wave transmission model of the umbilicoplacental circulation based on hemodynamic measurements in sheep.* Am J Physiol, 1995. 269(5 Pt 2): p. R1267-78.

709. Guiot, C., P.G. Pianta, and T. Todros, *Modelling the feto-placental circulation: 1. A distributed network predicting umbilical haemodynamics throughout pregnancy.* Ultrasound Med Biol, 1992. 18(6-7): p. 535-44.

710. Iwamoto, H.S., E. Stucky, and C.M. Roman, *Effect of graded umbilical cord compression in fetal sheep at 0.6, 0.7 gestation.* Am J Physiol, 1991. 261 (4 Pt 2): p. H1268-74.

711. Wilkening, R.B., *Effect of Occluding one umbilical artery on placental oxygen transport.* Am J Physiol 1991. 260(4(Pt 2)): p. H1319-25.

712. Frasch, M.G., et al., *Measures of acidosis with repetitive umbilical cord occlusions leading to fetal asphyxia in the near-term ovine fetus.* Am J Obstet Gynecol, 2009. 200(2): p. 200 e1-7.

713. Itskovitz, J., E.F. LaGamma, and A.M. Rudolph, *Effects of cord compression on fetal blood flow distribution and O2 delivery.* Am J Physiol, 1987. 252(1 Pt 2): p. H100-9.

714. Canavan, T.P., H.N. Simhan, and S. Caritis, *An evidence-based approach to the evaluation and treatment of premature rupture of membranes: Part I.* Obstet Gynecol Surv, 2004. 59(9): p. 669-77.

715. Rogers, M.S., et al., *Oxidative stress in the fetal lamb brain following intermittent umbilical cord occlusion: a path analysis.* BJOG, 2001. 108(12): p. 1283-90.

716. Wolfberg, A.J., et al., *Identification of fetal cerebral lactate using magnetic resonance spectroscopy.* Am J Obstet Gynecol, 2007. 196(1): p. e9-11.

717. Wolfberg, A.J. and E.R. Norwitz, *Probing the fetal cardiac signal for antecedents of brain injury.* Clin Perinatol, 2009. 36(3): p. 673-84.

718. Cottle, M.K., G.R. van Petten, and P. van Muyden, *Depression of uterine blood flow in response to cord compression in sheep.* Can J Physiol Pharmacol, 1982. 60(6): p. 825-9.

719. Hasaart, T.H. and J. de Haan, *Depression of uterine blood flow during total umbilical cord occlusion in sheep.* Eur J Obstet Gynecol Reprod Biol, 1985. 19(2): p. 125-31.

720. Robinson, K.S., R.J. Kavlock, and W.P. Watkinson, *Electrocardiographic responses of rat fetuses with clamped or intact umbilical cords to acute maternal uterine ischemia.* Am J Obstet Gynecol, 1983. 147(7): p. 795-8.

721. Millicovsky, G. and J.M. DeSesso, *Differential embryonic cardiovascular responses to acute maternal uterine ischemia: an in vivo microscopic study of rabbit embryos with either intact or clamped umbilical cords.* Teratology, 1980. 22(3): p. 335-43.

722. Kiserud, T., *Hemodynamics of the ductus venosus.* Eur J Obstet Gynecol Reprod Biol, 1999. 84(2): p. 139-47.

723. Hanson, M. and T. Kiserud, *Cardiovascular System*. Fetal growth and development, ed. R. Harding and A.D. Bocking. 2001, pg 70-93: Cambridge University Press.

724. Pennell, C.E., et al., *et al. Predictors of Physiologic and Histologic Responses to Repeated Cord Occlusion in the Near Term Ovine Fetus*. Fetal and Neonatal Physiologic Society 28th Annual Meeting Abstract, 2001: p. 93.

725. Rudolph, C.D., C. Roman, and A.M. Rudolph, *Effect of acute umbilical cord compression on hepatic carbohydrate metabolism in the fetal lamb*. Pediatr Res, 1989. 25(3): p. 228-33.

726. de Haan, H.H., A.J. Gunn, and P.D. Gluckman, *Fetal heart rate changes do not reflect cardiovascular deterioration during brief repeated umbilical cord occlusions in near-term fetal lambs*. Am J Obstet Gynecol, 1997. 176(1 Pt 1): p. 8-17.

727. Westgate, J.A., et al., *ST waveform changes during repeated umbilical cord occlusion in near-term fetal sheep*. Am J Obstet Gynecol, 2001. 184: p. 743-51.

728. Westgate, J.A., et al., *Fetal heart rate overshoot during repeated umbilical cord occlusion in sheep*. Obstet Gynecol, 2001. 97(3): p. 454-9.

729. Giussani, D.A., S.J.A. D., and M.A. Hanson, *Fetal cardiovascular reflex responses to hypoxaemia*. Fetal and Maternal Medicine Review, 1994. 6: p. 17-37.

730. Giussani, D.A., et al., *Dynamics of cardiovascular responses to repeated partial umbilical cord compression in late-gestation sheep fetus*. Am J Physiol, 1997. 273(5 Pt 2): p. H2351-60.

731. Jensen, A., Y. Garnier, and R. Berger, *Dynamics of fetal circulatory responses to hypoxia and asphyxia*. Eur J Obstet Gynecol Reprod Biol, 1999. 84(2): p. 155-72.

732. Tagiev, S.K., P.L. Dzhangirov, and K.B. Mamedov, *Bioelectric activity of the brain in rabbit fetuses in relation to the duration of umbilical cord occlusion*. Zh Evol Biokhim Fiziol, 1985. 21: p. 49-54.

733. Westgate, J.A., L. Bennet, and A.J. Gunn, *Intrapartum hypoxia*. Current Issues in Fetal and Neonatal Asphyxia Brain Injury, ed. S.M. Donn, S.K. Sinha, and M.L. Chiswick. 2001: 243-278, N.Y., N.Y.: Futura Publishing Co.

734. Phelan, J.P., *Advanced Fetal Monitoring 2001 and Legal Implications Symposium*, Medical Intelligence Co.: Pasadena, CA.

735. Maulik, D., *Asphyxia and Fetal Brain Damage*. 1998, N.Y., N.Y.: Wiley-Liss Publ.

736. Gualandri, G., et al., *Spontaneous umbilical cord hematoma: an unusual cause of fetal mortality: a report of 3 cases and review of the literature*. Am J Forensic Med Pathol, 2008. 29(2): p. 185-90.

737. Mendenhall, H.W., J.A. O'Leary, and K.O. Phillips, *The nonstress test: the value of a single acceleration in evaluating the fetus at risk*. Am J Obstet Gynecol, 1980. 136(1): p. 87-91.

738. Hon, E.H., *FETAL HEART RATE MONITORING*. Biomed Sci Instrum, 1963. 1: p. 287-91.

739. Hon, E.H., *Electronic evaluation of the fetal heart rate. VI. Fetal distress-a working hypothesis*. Am J Obstet Gynecol, 1962. 83: p. 333-53.

740. Cabaniss, M.L. and M.G. Ross, eds. *Fetal Monitoring Interpretation*. Second Edition ed. 2010, Lippincott Williams & Wilkins: Philadephia. 501.

741. Yeh, S.Y., et al., *Intrapartum fetal cardiac arrest. A preliminary observation*. Obstet Gynecol, 1977. 50(5): p. 571-7.

742. Lenke, R.R. and S. Trupin, *Sudden, unforeseen fetal death in a woman being treated for premature labor. A case report*. J Reprod Med, 1984. 29(12): p. 872-4.

743. Dellinger, E.H., F.H. Boehm, and M.M. Crane, *Electronic fetal heart rate monitoring: early neonatal outcomes associated with normal rate, fetal stress, and fetal distress*. Am J Obstet Gynecol, 2000. 182(1 Pt 1): p. 214-20.

744. Rubinstein, T.H. and B.S. Schifrin, *Decreased fetal movement with abnormal nonstress test preceding fetal death*. J Perinatol, 1992. 12(3): p. 294-6.

745. Kunzel, W. and B. Misselwitz, *Unexpected fetal death during pregnancy--a problem of unrecognized fetal disorders during antenatal care?* Eur J Obstet Gynecol Reprod Biol, 2003. 110 Suppl 1: p. S86-92.

746. Lamvu, G.M., et al., *Impact of abnormal results of outpatient fetal heart rate monitoring on maternal intervention in labor*. J Reprod Med, 2006. 51(9): p. 689-93.

747. Visser, G.H., D.J. Bekedam, and L.S. Ribbert, *Changes in antepartum heart rate patterns with progressive deterioration of the fetal condition*. Int J Biomed Comput, 1990. 25(4): p. 239-46.

748. Petrikovsky, B.M. and G.P. Kaplan, *Diurnal non-stress test variations in healthy term fetuses. A call for evening*

appointments for fetal testing. Early Hum Dev, 1996. 44(2): p. 127-30.

749. Genest, D.R., M.A. Williams, and M.F. Greene, *Estimating the time of death in stillborn fetuses: I. Histologic evaluation of fetal organs; an autopsy study of 150 stillborns.* Obstet Gynecol, 1992. 80(4): p. 575-84.

750. Babazadeh, R., et al., *Diurnal nonstress test variations in the human fetus at risk.* Int J Gynaecol Obstet, 2005. 90(3): p. 189-92.

751. Devoe, L.D., et al., *Clinical sequelae of the extended nonstress test.* Am J Obstet Gynecol, 1985. 151(8): p. 1074-8.

752. Bourgeois, F.J., S. Thiagarajah, and G.M. Harbert, Jr., *The significance of fetal heart rate decelerations during nonstress testing.* Am J Obstet Gynecol, 1984. 150(2): p. 213-6.

753. Izquierdo Puente, J.C., et al., *[Cardiotocography in intrauterine growth retardation].* Ginecol Obstet Mex, 1989. 57: p. 3-7.

754. Weber, S., et al., *[Antenatal fetal heart rate with special reference to maternal posture].* Geburtshilfe Frauenheilkd, 1988. 48(1): p. 35-40.

755. Cito, G., et al., *Maternal position during non-stress test and fetal heart rate patterns.* Acta Obstet Gynecol Scand, 2005. 84(4): p. 335-8.

756. Bourgin, C., et al., *[Perinatal pathology after normal pregnancies (author's transl)].* J Gynecol Obstet Biol Reprod (Paris), 1980. 9(6): p. 687-93.

757. Phelan, J.P., A.D. Cromartie, and C.V. Smith, *The nonstress test: the false negative test.* Am J Obstet Gynecol, 1982. 142(3): p. 293-6.

758. Barss, V.A., F.D. Frigoletto, and F. Diamond, *Stillbirth after nonstress testing.* Obstet Gynecol, 1985. 65(4): p. 541-4.

759. Freeman, R.K., G. Anderson, and W. Dorchester, *A prospective multi-institutional study of antepartum fetal heart rate monitoring. I. Risk of perinatal mortality and morbidity according to antepartum fetal heart rate test results.* Am J Obstet Gynecol, 1982. 143(7): p. 771-7.

760. Vintzileos, A.M., *Antenatal assessment for the detection of fetal asphyxia. An evidence-based approach using indication-specific testing.* Ann N Y Acad Sci, 2000. 900: p. 137-50.

761. Kontopoulos, E.V. and A.M. Vintzileos, *Condition-specific antepartum fetal testing.* Am J Obstet Gynecol, 2004. 191(5): p. 1546-51.

762. Phelan, J.P. and M.O. Ahn, *Fetal Heart Rate Observations in 300 Term Brain-damaged Infants.* J Matern Fetal Investig, 1998. 8(1): p. 1-5.

763. Salamalekis, E., et al., *Non-stress test: a fifteen-year clinical appraisal.* Clin Exp Obstet Gynecol, 1997. 24(2): p. 79-81.

764. Boehm, F.H., et al., *Improved outcome of twice weekly nonstress testing.* Obstet Gynecol, 1986. 67(4): p. 566-8.

765. Weeks, J.W., et al., *Antepartum surveillance for a history of stillbirth: when to begin?* Am J Obstet Gynecol, 1995. 172(2 Pt 1): p. 486-92.

766. Miller, D.A., *Antepartum testing.* Clin Obstet Gynecol, 1998. 41(3): p. 647-53.

767. Pattison, N. and L. McCowan, *Cardiotocography for antepartum fetal assessment.* Cochrane Database Syst Rev, 2000(2): p. CD001068.

768. Flynn, A.M., et al., *A randomized controlled trial of non-stress antepartum cardiotocography.* Br J Obstet Gynaecol, 1982. 89(6): p. 427-33.

769. Quemere, M.P., et al., *[Fetal home telemonitoring: the Nancy experience from 1992-1997. analysis of 12649 recordings].* J Gynecol Obstet Biol Reprod (Paris), 2000. 29(6): p. 571-8.

770. Meystre, S., *The current state of telemonitoring: a comment on the literature.* Telemed J E Health, 2005. 11(1): p. 63-9.

771. Salomon, L.J., et al., *Fetal home monitoring for the prenatal management of gastroschisis.* Acta Obstet Gynecol Scand, 2004. 83(11): p. 1061-4.

772. Kerner, R., et al., *Maternal self-administered fetal heart rate monitoring and transmission from home in high-risk pregnancies.* Int J Gynaecol Obstet, 2004. 84(1): p. 33-9.

773. Hod, M. and R. Kerner, *Telemedicine for antenatal surveillance of high-risk pregnancies with ambulatory and home fetal heart rate monitoring--an update.* J Perinat Med, 2003. 31(3): p. 195-200.

774. Pan, J., et al., *[Value of long-distance fetal heart rate monitoring on the pre-partum health care of the pregnant woman with umbilical cord loops].* Zhonghua Fu Chan Ke Za Zhi, 2002. 37(8): p. 451-4.

775. Naef, R.W., 3rd, et al., *Assessment of fetal well-being using the nonstress test in the home setting.* Obstet Gynecol, 1994. 84(3): p. 424-6.

776. Duminy, P.C. and L. October, *Telemetric antenatal fetal monitoring.* S Afr Med J, 2005. 95(4): p. 250-2.

777. Budinger, T.F., *Biomonitoring with wireless communications.* Annu Rev Biomed Eng, 2003. 5: p. 383-412.

778. Dawson, A., et al., *Domiciliary midwifery support in high-risk pregnancy incorporating telephonic fetal heart rate monitoring: a health technology randomized assessment.* J Telemed Telecare, 1999. 5(4): p. 220-30.

779. Horio, H., et al., *Fetal monitor for non-stress-test screening at home.* Biomed Instrum Technol, 1998. 32(1): p. 39-47.

780. Horio, H., et al., *Clinical telecommunication network system for home monitoring.* Med Biol Eng Comput, 1994. 32(2): p. 227-30.

781. Barbarino-Monnier, P., et al., *[Importance of fetal cardiac rhythm monitoring at home in the follow-up of pregnancies at risk: evaluation following 2 years of utilization].* Rev Med Liege, 1992. 47(9): p. 461-9.

782. Gonen, R., N. Braithwaite, and J.E. Milligan, *Fetal heart rate monitoring at home and transmission by telephone.* Obstet Gynecol, 1990. 75(3 Pt 1): p. 464-8.

783. Su, F. and X. Guo, *[Clinical application of the expert type terminal of remote electronic fetal heart rate home monitoring system].* Zhonghua Fu Chan Ke Za Zhi, 2002. 37(8): p. 459-61.

784. Acker, D.B., et al., *The nonstress test. Transmission from the home.* J Reprod Med, 1989. 34(12): p. 971-4.

785. Reece, E.A., et al., *A controlled trial of self-nonstress test versus assisted nonstress test in the evaluation of fetal well-being.* Am J Obstet Gynecol, 1992. 166(2): p. 489-92.

786. Kitagawa, M., et al., *Development and clinical application of a telemedicine support system in the field of perinatal patient management.* J Obstet Gynaecol Res, 2000. 26(6): p. 427-34.

787. Warland, J., H. McCutcheon, and P. Baghurst, *Maternal blood pressure in pregnancy and stillbirth: a case-control study of third-trimester stillbirth.* Am J Perinatol, 2008. 25(5): p. 311-7.

788. Lalor, J.G., et al., *Biophysical profile for fetal assessment in high risk pregnancies.* Cochrane Database Syst Rev, 2008(1): p. CD000038.

789. Walker, C. and J. Ward, *Intrapartum umbilical cord rupture.* Obstet Gynecol, 2009. 113(2 Pt 2): p. 552-4.

790. Tsafrir, A. and Y. Shufaro, *A fatal true knot of cord.* J Obstet Gynaecol Can, 2008. 30(11): p. 993, 994.

791. Burke, C.J. and A.E. Tannenberg, *Intrapartum stillbirths in hospital unrelated to uteroplacental vascular insufficiency.* Pediatr Dev Pathol, 2007. 10(1): p. 35-40.

792. Osawa, K., et al., *A case of fetal vesicoallantoic cyst in the umbilical cord.* Fetal Diagn Ther, 2003. 18(2): p. 87-90.

793. Pommerenke, F. and W. Sadenwasser, *[Umbilical cord compression by an amnionic band].* Zentralbl Gynakol, 1992. 114(11): p. 557-9.

794. Shipp, T.D., B. Bromley, and B.R. Benacerraf, *Sonographically detected abnormalities of the umbilical cord.* Int J Gynaecol Obstet, 1995. 48(2): p. 179-85.

795. Battaglia, C., et al., *Cord vessel compression by an expanding allantoic cyst: case report.* Ultrasound Obstet Gynecol, 1992. 2(1): p. 58-60.

796. Shenker, L., W. Anderson, and C. Anderson, *Ultrasound demonstration of masses in a 15 week fetus: hydrops in a fetus with umbilical cord occlusion.* Prenat Diagn, 1981. 1(3): p. 217-21.

797. Rocha, E., R. Hammond, and B. Richardson, *Necrotic cell injury in the preterm and near-term ovine fetal brain after intermittent umbilical cord occlusion.* Am J Obstet Gynecol, 2004. 191(2): p. 488-96.

798. Sepulveda, W., et al., *Fetal death due to umbilical cord hematoma: a rare complication of umbilical cord cyst.* J Matern Fetal Neonatal Med, 2005. 18(6): p. 387-90.

799. Brown, R. and K. Nicolaides, *Umbilical cord hematoma associated with an umbilical cord cyst and fetal death at 28 weeks of gestation.* J Ultrasound Med, 2000. 19(3): p. 223-5.

800. Papadopoulos, V.G., et al., *A case of umbilical cord hemangioma: Doppler studies and review of the literature.* Eur J Obstet Gynecol Reprod Biol, 2009. 144(1): p. 8-14.

801. Makhoul, I.R., et al., *[Spontaneous umbilical cord hematoma].* Harefuah, 2005. 144(4): p. 237-8, 304.

802. Sizun, J., et al., *[Spontaneous umbilical cord hematoma, a rare cause of acute fetal distress].* Arch Pediatr, 1995. 2(12): p. 1182-3.

803. Feldberg, D., et al., *Hematoma of the umbilical cord with acute antepartum fetal distress. A case report.* J Reprod Med, 1986. 31(1): p. 65-6.

804. Ottolenghi-Preti, G.F., L. Magnani, and A. Paghera, *[Umbilical cord hematoma. 2 case reports and review of the literature].* Ann Ostet Ginecol Med Perinat, 1972. 93(8): p. 562-78.

805. Naidu, M., et al., *Umbilical cord rupture: a case report and review of literature.* Int J Fertil Womens Med, 2007. 52(2-3): p. 107-10.

806. Summerville, J.W., J.S. Powar, and K. Ueland, *Umbilical cord hematoma resulting in intrauterine fetal demise. A case report.* J Reprod Med, 1987. 32(3): p. 213-6.

807. Heifetz, S.A., *Thrombosis of the umbilical cord: analysis of 52 cases and literature review.* Pediatr Pathol, 1988. 8(1): p. 37-54.

808. Vougiouklakis, T., et al., *Ruptured hemangioma of the umbilical cord and intrauterine fetal death, with review data.* Pathol Res Pract, 2006. 202(7): p. 537-40.

809. Panda, B., et al., *Prenatal diagnosis of an umbilical vein aneurysm: a case report.* Conn Med, 2009. 73(8): p. 465-7.

810. Sato, Y. and K. Benirschke, *Umbilical arterial thrombosis with vascular wall necrosis: clinicopathologic findings of 11 cases.* Placenta, 2006. 27(6-7): p. 715-8.

811. Klaritsch, P., et al., *Spontaneous intrauterine umbilical artery thrombosis leading to severe fetal growth restriction.* Placenta, 2008. 29(4): p. 374-7.

812. Sepulveda, W., *Umbilical artery aneurysm:Prenatal identification in three fetuses with trisomy.* Ultrasound Obstet Gynecol, 2003. 21: p. 213-4.

813. Shen, O., *Prenatal Diagnosis of umbilical artery aneurysm.* J Ultrasound Med, 2007. 26: p. 251-3.

814. Fung, T.Y., *Fetal intra-abdominal umbilical vein varix what: what is the clinical significance?* Ultrasound Obstet Gynecol 2005. 25: p. 149-54.

815. Miyake, H., et al., *Umbilical cord ulceration after prenatal diagnosis of duodenal atresia with interstitial deletion of chromosome 13q: a case report.* Fetal Diagn Ther, 2008. 24(2): p. 115-8.

816. Anami, A., et al., *Sudden fetal death associated with both duodenal atresia and umbilical cord ulcer: a case report and review.* Am J Perinatol, 2006. 23(3): p. 183-8.

817. Kimura, T., et al., *Umbilical cord ulcer associated with fetal jejunal atresia: report of 2 cases.* Fetal Diagn Ther, 2003. 18(3): p. 144-7.

818. Nijagal, A., et al., *Intrauterine umbilical cord hemorrhage with associated jejunal atresia captured by real-time ultrasound.* Am J Obstet Gynecol, 2009. 200(3): p. e5-6.

819. Yamanaka, M., et al., *Umbilical cord ulceration and intestinal atresia.* Eur J Obstet Gynecol Reprod Biol, 1996. 70(2): p. 209-12.

820. Altshuler, G., M. Arizawa, and G. Molnar-Nadasdy, *Meconium-induced umbilical cord vascular necrosis and ulceration: a potential link between the placenta and poor pregnancy outcome.* Obstet Gynecol, 1992. 79(5 (Pt 1)): p. 760-6.

821. Sienko, A. and G. Altshuler, *Meconium-induced umbilical vascular necrosis in abortuses and fetuses: a histopathologic study for cytokines.* Obstet Gynecol, 1999. 94(3): p. 415-20.

822. Park, J.Y., et al., *Comparative proteomic analysis of malformed umbilical cords from somatic cell nuclear transfer-derived piglets: implications for early postnatal death.* BMC Genomics, 2009. 10(1): p. 511.

823. Soong, Y.K., et al., *Genome-wide detection of uniparental disomy in a fetus with intrauterine growth restriction using genotyping microarrays.* Taiwan J Obstet Gynecol, 2009. 48(2): p. 152-8.

824. Sanchez, J.M., et al., *Severe fetal malformations associated with trisomy 16 confined to the placenta.* Prenat Diagn, 1997. 17(8): p. 777-9.

825. Fleischer AC, e.a., ed. *Sonography and Obstetrics and Gynecology.* Sixth ed. Sonography of the Umbilical Cord. 2001, McGraw-Hill: USA. 225-245.

826. Vayssiere, C., et al., *Diagnosing umbilical cord entanglement in monoamniotic twins: becoming easier and probably essential.* Ultrasound Obstet Gynecol, 2004. 24(5): p. 587-9.

827. Bernholtz, J.C., *Ecologic physiology of the fetus. Ultrasonography of supply-line deprivation syndromes.* Radiol Clin North Amer, 1990. 28: p. 179-88.

828. Nelson, L.H., *Ultrasonography of the Placenta - A Review.* 1994 AIUM, Rockville, MD: American Institute of Ultrasound in Medicine.

829. Hill, L.M., S. Kislak, and C. Runco, *An ultrasonic view of the umbilical cord.* Obstet Gynecol Surv, 1987. 42(2): p. 82-8.

830. Sherer, D.M. and A. Anyaegbunam, *Prenatal ultrasonographic morphologic assessment of the umbilical cord: a review. Part I.* Obstet Gynecol Surv, 1997. 52(8): p. 506-14.

831. Sherer, D.M. and A. Anyaegbunam, *Prenatal ultrasonographic morphologic assessment of the umbilical cord: a review. Part II.* Obstet Gynecol Surv, 1997. 52(8): p. 515-23.

832. Kurjak, A., ed. *Three-Dimensional Power Doppler in Obstetrics and Gynecology.* 2000, Parthenon Publishing: N.Y., N.Y.

833. Harris, R.D. and R.D. Alexander, *Ultrasound of the Placenta and Umbilical Cord.* Ultrasonography in Obstetrics and Gynecology (ed 4), ed. P.W. Callen. 2000, Philadelphia, PA: W B Saunders Co.

834. Kinare, A., *Fetal environment.* Indian J Radiol Imaging, 2008. 18(4): p. 326-44.

835. Sepulveda, W., et al., *Improving sonographic evaluation of the umbilical cord at the second-trimester anatomy scan.* J Ultrasound Med, 2009. 28(6): p. 831-5.

836. Henrich, W. and B. Tutschek, *Cord entanglement in monoamniotic twins: 2D and 3D colour Doppler studies.* Ultraschall Med, 2008. 29 Suppl 5: p. 271-2.

837. Chen, Q.K. and L.R. Tian, *[Diagnostic value of ultrasound in fetal umbilical cord coiling around the head: report of 3 cases].* Di Yi Jun Yi Da Xue Xue Bao, 2005. 25(6): p. 671.

838. Perlitz, Y., *Acute polyhydramnios in term pregnancy may be caused by multiple nuchal loops.* Ultrasound Obstet Gynecol, 2010. 35: p. 253-4.

839. Morin, F.R. and F. Winsberg, *The ultrasonic appearance of the umbilical cord.* J Clin Ultrasound, 1978. 6(5): p. 324-6.

840. Jauniaux, E., et al., *Correlation of ultrasound and pathologic findings of placental anomalies in pregnancies with elevated maternal serum alpha-fetoprotein.* Eur J Obstet Gynecol Reprod Biol, 1990. 37(3): p. 219-30.

841. Thompson, R.S., B.J. Trudinger, and C.M. Cook, *A comparison of Doppler ultrasound waveform indices in the umbilical artery--I. Indices derived from the maximum velocity waveform.* Ultrasound Med Biol, 1986. 12(11): p. 835-44.

842. Jauniaux, E., S. Campbell, and S. Vyas, *The use of color Doppler imaging for prenatal diagnosis of umbilical cord anomalies: report of three cases.* Am J Obstet Gynecol, 1989. 161: p. 1195-7.

843. Sohaey, R., *Amniotic fluid and the umbilical cord: the fetal milieu and lifeline.* Semin Ultrasound CT MR, 1998. 19(4): p. 355-69.

844. Weissman, A. and P. Jakobi, *Sonographic measurements of the umbilical cord in pregnancies complicated by gestational diabetes.* J Ultrasound Med, 1997. 16(10): p. 691-4.

845. Dudiak, C.M., et al., *Sonography of the umbilical cord.* Radiographics, 1995. 15(5): p. 1035-50.

846. Hata, T., et al., *Three-dimensional ultrasonographic assessment of the umbilical cord during the 2nd and 3rd trimesters of pregnancy.* Gynecol Obstet Invest, 1998. 45(3): p. 159-64.

847. Sherer, D.M. and F.A. Manning, *Prenatal ultrasonographic diagnosis of conditions associated with potential umbilical cord compression.* Am J Perinatol, 1999. 16(9): p. 445-58.

848. Woodward, P.M., et al., ed. *Diagnostic Imaging.* First ed. Obstetrics. Vol. I. 2005, AMIRSYS: Salt Lake City. CH 11, 25.

849. Raio, L., et al., *Prenatal diagnosis of a lean umbilical cord: a simple marker for the fetus at risk of being small for gestational age at birth.* Ultrasound Obstet Gynecol, 1999. 13(3): p. 176-80.

850. Hill, L.M., D.M. DiNofrio, and D. Guzick, *Sonographic determination of first trimester umbilical cord length.* J Clin Ultrasound, 1994. 22(7): p. 435-8.

851. Collins, J.H., *Ultrasound measurement of umbilical cord length.* J Ultrasound Med, 1994. 13(11): p. 854.

852. Funk, A., L. Verstraete, and A. Gans, *Vaginal sonographic diagnosis of the missing umbilical cord syndrome.* Z Geburtshilfe Perinatol, 1991. 195: p. 54-6.

853. Hill, L.M., et al., *Persistent right umbilical vein: sonographic detection and subsequent neonatal outcome.* Obstet Gynecol, 1994. 84(6): p. 923-5.

854. Hamanda, H., et al., *Prenatal sonographic diagnosis of Beck-Weidemann syndrome in association with a single umbilical artery.* J Clin Ultrasound, 2001. 29: p. 535-38.

855. Jassani, M.N., J.N. Brennan, and I.R. Merkatz, *Prenatal diagnosis of single umbilical artery by ultrasound.* J Clin Ultrasound, 1980. 8(5): p. 447-8.

856. Rosenak, D. and I. Meizner, *Prenatal sonographic detection of single and double umbilical artery in the same fetus.* J Ultrasound Med, 1994. 13(12): p. 995-6.

857. Kinare, A.S., et al., *Prenatal diagnosis with ultrasound of anomalous course of the umbilical vein and its relationship to fetal outcome.* J Clin Ultrasound, 1996. 24(7): p. 333-8.

858. Hill, L.M., et al., *Validity of transabdominal sonography in the detection of a two-vessel umbilical cord.* Obstet Gynecol, 2001. 98(5 Pt 1): p. 837-42.

859. Hitschold, T. and H. Muntefering, *[Single umbilical artery. Effect on fetal growth and doppler flow velocity wave form].* Ultraschall Med, 2001. 22(1): p. 17-22.

860. Raga, F., et al., *Role of color flow Doppler ultrasonography in diagnosing velamentous insertion of the umbilical cord*

and vasa previa. A report of two cases. J Reprod Med, 1995. 40(11): p. 804-8.

861. Nomiyama, M., Y. Toyota, and H. Kawano, *Antenatal diagnosis of velamentous umbilical cord insertion and vasa previa with color Doppler imaging.* Ultrasound Obstet Gynecol, 1998. 12(6): p. 426-9.

862. Monteagudo, A., A.K. Sfakianaki, and I.E. Timor-Tritsch, *Velamentous insertion of the cord in the first trimester.* Ultrasound Obstet Gynecol, 2000. 16(5): p. 498-9.

863. Daly-Jones, E., J. Hollingsworth, and W. Sepulveda, *Vasa praevia: second trimester diagnosis using colour flow imaging.* Br J Obstet Gynaecol, 1996. 103(3): p. 284-6.

864. Lee, W., et al., *Vasa previa: prenatal diagnosis, natural evolution, and clinical outcome.* Obstet Gynecol, 2000. 95(4): p. 572-6.

865. Hertzberg, B.S. and M.A. Kliewer, *Vasa previa: prenatal diagnosis by transperineal sonography with Doppler evaluation.* J Clin Ultrasound, 1998. 26(8): p. 405-8.

866. Baschat, A.A. and U. Gembruch, *Ante- and intrapartum diagnosis of vasa praevia in singleton pregnancies by colour coded Doppler sonography.* Eur J Obstet Gynecol Reprod Biol, 1998. 79(1): p. 19-25.

867. Oyelese, K.O., et al., *Vasa previa: an avoidable obstetric tragedy.* Obstet Gynecol Surv, 1999. 54(2): p. 138-45.

868. Christopher, C.R., A. Spinelli, and M.L. Collins, *Ultrasonic detection of "hourglass membranes" with funic presentation.* Obstet Gynecol, 1979. 54(1): p. 130-2.

869. Vintzileos, A.M., et al., *Ultrasonic diagnosis of funic presentation.* J Clin Ultrasound, 1983. 11(9): p. 510-1.

870. Jurgens, J. and J. Woll, *[Theoretical and experimental models of sonographic diagnosis of umbilical cord knot and their application in practice]*. Z Geburtshilfe Neonatol, 1999. 203(2): p. 73-6.

871. Collins, J.H., *First report: prenatal diagnosis of a true knot.* Am J Obstet Gynecol, 1991. 165(6 Pt 1): p. 1898.

872. Hertzberg, B.S., et al., *False knot of the umbilical cord: sonographic appearance and differential diagnosis.* J Clin Ultrasound, 1988. 16(8): p. 599-602.

873. Jeanty, P., *Fetal and funicular vascular anomalies: identification with prenatal US.* Radiology, 1989. 173(2): p. 367-70.

874. Jouppila, P. and P. Kirkinen, *Ultrasonic diagnosis of nuchal encirclement by the umbilical cord: a case and methodological report.* J Clin Ultrasound, 1982. 10(2): p. 59-62.

875. Verdel, M.J. and N. Exalto, *Tight nuchal coiling of the umbilical cord causing fetal death.* J Clin Ultrasound, 1994. 22(1): p. 64-6.

876. Ranzini, A.C., C.A. Walters, and A.M. Vintzileos, *Ultrasound diagnosis of nuchal cord: the gray-scale divot sign.* Obstet Gynecol, 1999. 93(5 Pt 2): p. 854.

877. Shukunami, K. and F. Kotsuji, *Nuchal cord position in breech presentation: case report.* J Matern Fetal Med, 2000. 9(2): p. 153-4.

878. Morgan-Ortiz, F., et al., *[Evaluation of ultrasound as a diagnostic test in nuchal encirclement by the umbilical cord during labor].* Ginecol Obstet Mex, 1997. 65: p. 529-32.

879. Tongsong, T. and P. Chanprapaph, *Picture of the month. Evolution of umbilical cord entanglement in monoamniotic twins.* Ultrasound Obstet Gynecol, 1999. 14(1): p. 75-7.

880. De Lia, J.E. and D. Worthington, *Intrauterine sling with umbilical cord entanglement in diamniotic twins.* Ultrasound Obstet Gynecol, 2000. 15(5): p. 447.

881. Abrams, S.L., P.W. Callen, and R.A. Filly, *Umbilical vein thrombosis: sonographic detection in utero.* J Ultrasound Med, 1985. 4(6): p. 283-5.

882. Allen, S.L., et al., *Thrombosing umbilical vein varix.* J Ultrasound Med, 1998. 17(3): p. 189-92.

883. Afriat, R., et al., *[Prenatal diagnosis of spontaneous thrombosis of the umbilical artery during the third trimester of pregnancy. Two cases with surviving infants].* J Gynecol Obstet Biol Reprod (Paris), 1995. 24(4): p. 411-4.

884. Sepulveda, W., et al., *Pseudocyst of the umbilical cord: prenatal sonographic appearance and clinical significance.* Obstet Gynecol, 1999. 93(3): p. 377-81.

885. Sepulveda, W., et al., *Clinical significance of first trimester umbilical cord cysts.* J Ultrasound Med, 1999. 18(2): p. 95-9.

886. Skibo, L.K., E.A. Lyons, and C.S. Levi, *First-trimester umbilical cord cysts.* Radiology, 1992. 182(3): p. 719-22.

887. Petrikovsky, B.M., et al., *Prenatal diagnosis of non-iatrogenic hematoma of the umbilical cord.* J Clin Ultrasound, 1996. 24(1): p. 37-9.

888. Sepulveda, W., et al., *Discordant umbilical artery flow velocity waveforms in spontaneous umbilical cord hematoma.* J Clin Ultrasound, 1995. 23(5): p. 330-2.

889. Gregora, M.G. and J. Lai, *Umbilical cord haematoma: a serious pregnancy complication.* Aust N Z J Obstet Gynaecol, 1995. 35(2): p. 212-4.

890. Seifer, D.B., et al., *Nonimmune hydrops fetalis in association with hemangioma of the umbilical cord.* Obstet Gynecol, 1985. 66(2): p. 283-6.

891. Carles, D., et al., *[Lethal hydrops fetalis secondary to an umbilical cord hemangioma].* Ann Pathol, 1994. 14(4): p. 244-7.

892. Bruhwiler, H., M. Rabner, and K.P. Luscher, *Pranatle diagnose eines Nabelschnur: Hamangioms bei erhohtem Alpha fotoprotein.* Ultraschall Med, 1994. 15: p. 140.

893. Siddiqi, T.A., et al., *Umbilical artery aneurysm: prenatal diagnosis and management.* Obstet Gynecol, 1992. 80(3 Pt 2): p. 530-3.

894. Berg, C., et al., *Prenatal diagnosis of umbilical cord aneurysm in a fetus with trisomy 18.* Ultrasound Obstet Gynecol, 2001. 17(1): p. 79-81.

895. Vandevijver, N., et al., *Aneurysm of the umbilical vein: case report and review of literature.* Eur J Obstet Gynecol Reprod Biol, 2000. 89(1): p. 85-7.

896. Rahemtullah, A., et al., *Outcome of pregnancy after prenatal diagnosis of umbilical vein varix.* J Ultrasound Med, 2001. 20(2): p. 135-9.

897. Estroff, J.A. and B.R. Benacerraf, *Fetal umbilical vein varix: sonographic appearance and postnatal outcome.* J Ultrasound Med, 1992. 11(3): p. 69-73.

898. Tennstedt, C., et al., *Angiomyxoma of the umbilical cord in one twin with cystic degeneration of Wharton's jelly. A case report.* Pathol Res Pract, 1998. 194(1): p. 55-8.

899. Wilson, R.D., et al., *In utero decompression of umbilical cord angiomyxoma followed by vaginal delivery.* Am J Obstet Gynecol, 1994. 171(5): p. 1383-5.

900. Gramellini, D., et al., *Color Doppler ultrasound in prenatal diagnosis of umbilical cord angiomyxoma. Case report.* Clin Exp Obstet Gynecol, 1993. 20(4): p. 241-4.

901. Satge, D.C., et al., *An umbilical cord teratoma in a 17-week-old fetus.* Prenat Diagn, 2001. 21(4): p. 284-8.

902. Kanayama, M.D., T.A. Gaffey, and P.L. Ogburn, Jr., *Constriction of the umbilical cord by an amniotic band, with fetal compromise illustrated by reverse diastolic flow in the umbilical artery. A case report.* J Reprod Med, 1995. 40(1): p. 71-3.

903. Lee, W., et al., *Vasa previa: prenatal detection by three-dimensional ultrasonography.* Ultrasound Obstet Gynecol, 2000. 16(4): p. 384-7.

904. Shi, J.C. and F.J. Hsieh, *Implemented 3D power Doppler for the evaluation of fetal and placental circulation.* Frontiers in Fetal Medicine, 2001. 3: p. 228-46.

905. Showa, A., et al. *Antenatal dianosis of aberrant umbilical vessels.* Gynecol Obstet Invest, 1997. 43: p. 232-35.

906. Van Calsteren, K., et al., *Feasibility of ultrasound-guided percutaneous samplings in the pregnant baboon: a model for studies on transplacental transport.* Reprod Sci, 2009. 16(3): p. 280-5.

907. Tongprasert, F., et al., *Cordocentesis in multifetal pregnancies.* Prenat Diagn, 2007. 27(12): p. 1100-3.

908. Tongsong, T., et al., *Cordocentesis at 16-24 weeks of gestation: experience of 1,320 cases.* Prenat Diagn, 2000. 20(3): p. 224-8.

909. Liao, C., et al., *Efficacy and safety of cordocentesis for prenatal diagnosis.* Int J Gynaecol Obstet, 2006. 93(1): p. 13-7.

910. De Lia, J.E., *Surgery of the placenta and umbilical cord.* Clin Obstet Gynecol, 1996. 39(3): p. 607-25.

911. Quintero, R., et al., *[Fetal endoscopic surgery in a case of twin pregnancy complicated by reversed arterial perfusion sequence (TRAP sequence)].* Rev Chil Obstet Ginecol, 1995. 60(2): p. 112-6; discussion 116-7.

912. Quintero, R.A., et al., *Selective photocoagulation of communicating vessels in the treatment of monochorionic twins with selective growth retardation.* Am J Obstet Gynecol, 2001. 185(3): p. 689-96.

913. Peiro, J.L., et al., *Therapeutic indications of fetoscopy: a 5-year institutional experience.* J Laparoendosc Adv Surg Tech A, 2009. 19(2): p. 229-36.

914. Liao, H., et al., *Fast image mapping of endoscopic image mosaics with three-dimensional ultrasound image for intrauterine fetal surgery.* Minim Invasive Ther Allied Technol, 2009: p. 1-9.

915. Hopkins, L.M. and V.A. Feldstein, *The use of ultrasound in fetal surgery.* Clin Perinatol, 2009. 36(2): p. 255-72, viii.

916. Di Salvo, D.N., et al., *Sonographic evaluation of the placental cord insertion site.* AJR, 1998. 170: p. 1295-98.

917. Sepulveda, W., et al., *Prenatal detection of velamentous insertion of the umbilical cord: a prospective color Doppler ultrasound study.* Ultrasound Obstet Gynecol, 2003. 21(6): p. 564-9.

918. Nicolaides, K.H., G. Rizzo, and K. Hecher, *Placental and fetal Doppler.* 2000, N.Y., N.Y.: Parthenon Publishing.

919. Bruch, J.F., et al., *Computerized microscope morphometry of umbilical vessels from pregnancies with intrauterine growth retardation and abnormal umbilical artery Doppler.* Hum Pathol, 1997. 28(10): p. 1139-45.

920. Weissman, A. and A. Drugan, *Sonographic findings of the umbilical cord: implications for the risk of fetal chromosomal anomalies.* Ultrasound Obstet Gynecol, 2001. 17(6): p. 536-41.

921. Sepulveda, W., *Time for a more detailed prenatal examination of the umbilical cord?* Ultrasound Obstet Gynecol, 1999. 13(3): p. 157-60.

922. Sherer, D.M. and F.A. Manning, *Prenatal ultrasonographic diagnosis of nuchal cord(s): disregard, inform, monitor or intervene?* Ultrasound Obstet Gynecol, 1999. 14(1): p. 1-8.

923. Entezami, M., R. Vonk, and R. Becker, *Nuchal cord.* Ultrasound Obstet Gynecol, 1999. 14(5): p. 362-3.

924. Siassakos, D., et al., *Retrospective cohort study of diagnosis-delivery interval with umbilical cord prolapse: the effect of team training.* BJOG, 2009. 116(8): p. 1089-96.

925. Tan, W.C., et al., *Audit of 'crash' emergency caesarean sections due to cord prolapse in terms of response time and perinatal outcome.* Ann Acad Med Singapore, 2003. 32(5): p. 638-41.

926. Hamilton, S. and L. Byrd, *Cord entanglement and/or knotting: is this only a feature of monochorionic monoamniotic pregnancies?* J Obstet Gynaecol, 2009. 29(3): p. 244-5.

927. Grzesiak, M., et al., *[Umbilical cord entanglement in monoamniotic twin preganacy--case presentation and literature review]*. Ginekol Pol, 2006. 77(9): p. 720-5.

928. Arabin, B., R.N. Laurini, and J. van Eyck, *Early prenatal diagnosis of cord entanglement in monoamniotic multiple pregnancies.* Ultrasound Obstet Gynecol, 1999. 13(3): p. 181-6.

929. Merien, A.E., J. van Eyck, and B. Arabin, *Two cases with dichorionic diamniotic triplet pregnancy and early cord entanglement.* Twin Res, 2001. 4(4): p. 219-22.

930. Hagen-Ansert, S.L., ed. *Diagnostic Ultrasonography.* Sixth ed. The Umbilical Cord Ch 52. 2000, Mosby: New York. 1156-1168.

931. Marsal, K., *Abnormal antenatal ultrasound findings and subsequent handicap.* Baillieres Clin Obstet Gynaecol, 1988. 2(1): p. 125-44.

932. Zangen, R. and H. Yaffe, *[Umbilical cord cyst--should it concern us?].* Harefuah, 2009. 148(7): p. 436-40, 475.

933. Aisenbrey, G.A., et al., *Monoamniotic and pseudomonoamniotic twins: sonographic diagnosis, detection of cord entanglement, and obstetric management.* Obstet Gynecol, 1995. 86(2): p. 218-22.

934. Pasquini, L., et al., *High perinatal survival in monoamniotic twins managed by prophylactic sulindac, intensive ultrasound surveillance, and Cesarean delivery at 32 weeks' gestation.* Ultrasound Obstet Gynecol, 2006. 28(5): p. 681-7.

935. Dias, T., et al., *Cord entanglement and perinatal outcome in monoamniotic twin pregnancies.* Ultrasound Obstet Gynecol. 35(2): p. 201-4.

936. Giannopoulos, T., P. O'Brien, and R. Varma, *Successful delivery of monoamniotic triplets.* BJOG, 2001. 108(8): p. 892-4.

937. West, C.R., Y. Adi, and P.O. Pharoah, *Fetal and infant death in mono- and dizygotic twins in England and Wales 1982-91.* Arch Dis Child Fetal Neonatal Ed, 1999. 80(3): p. F217-20.

938. Belfort, M.A., et al., *The use of color flow Doppler ultrasonography to diagnose umbilical cord entanglement in monoamniotic twin gestations.* Am J Obstet Gynecol, 1993. 168(2): p. 601-4.

939. Victoria, A., G. Mora, and F. Arias, *Perinatal outcome, placental pathology, and severity of discordance in monochorionic and dichorionic twins.* Obstet Gynecol, 2001. 97(2): p. 310-5.

940. Rodis, J.F., et al., *Monoamniotic twins: improved perinatal survival with accurate prenatal diagnosis and antenatal fetal surveillance.* Am J Obstet Gynecol, 1997. 177(5): p. 1046-9.

941. Lyndrup, J. and L. Schouenborg, *Cord entanglement in monoamniotic twin pregnancies.* Eur J Obstet Gynecol Reprod Biol, 1987. 26(3): p. 275-8.

942. Beasley, E., et al., *Monoamniotic twins: case series and proposal for antenatal management.* Obstet Gynecol, 1999. 93(1): p. 130-4.

943. Ashis, K., S. Neales, and K. Neales, *Double survival despite cord intertwining in monoamniotic twins.* Acta Obstet Gynecol Scand, 2001. 80: p. 974-75.

944. Krussel, J.S., S. von Eckardstein, and T. Schwenzer, *[Double umbilical cord knot in mono-amniotic twin pregnancy as the cause of intrauterine fetal death of both twins].* Zentralbl Gynakol, 1994. 116(8): p. 497-9.

945. Overton, T.G., et al., *First-trimester cord entanglement in monoamniotic twins.* Ultrasound Obstet Gynecol, 1999. 13(2): p. 140-2.

946. Rosemond, R.L. and N.E. Hinds, *Persistent abnormal umbilical cord Doppler velocimetry in a monoamniotic twin with cord entanglement.* J Ultrasound Med, 1998. 17(5): p. 337-8.

947. Abuhamad, A.Z., et al., *Umbilical artery flow velocity waveforms in monoamniotic twins with cord entanglement.* Obstet Gynecol, 1995. 86(4 Pt 2): p. 674-7.

948. Suzuki, S., et al., *Umbilical venous pulsation indicating tight cord entanglement in monoamniotic twin pregnancy.* J Ultrasound Med, 1999. 18(6): p. 425-7.

949. Westover, T., E.R. Guzman, and S. Shen-Schwarz, *Prenatal diagnosis of an unusual nuchal cord complication in monoamniotic twins.* Obstet Gynecol, 1994. 84(4 Pt 2): p. 689-91.

950. Pinette, M.G., et al., *Diagnosis of monochorionic monoamniotic twins by color Doppler: case report.* J Mater Fetal Invest, 1994. 4: p. 191-193.

951. Shahabi, S., et al., *Monoamniotic twin cord entanglement. A case report with color flow Doppler Ultrasonography for antenatal diagnosis.* J Reprod Med, 1997. 42(11): p. 740-2.

952. Sau, A.K. and K. Neales, *Double survival despite cord intertwining in monoamniotic twins.* Acta Obstet Gynecol Scand, 2001. 80(10): p. 974-5.

953. Ritossa, M. and J. O'Loughlin, *Monoamniotic twin pregnancy and cord entanglement: a clinical dilemma.* Aust N Z J Obstet Gynaecol, 1996. 36(3): p. 309-12.

954. Allen, V.M., et al., *Management of monoamniotic twin pregnancies: a case series and systematic review of the literature.* BJOG, 2001. 108(9): p. 931-6.

955. Delbaere, I., et al., *Umbilical cord anomalies are more frequent in twins after assisted reproduction.* Hum Reprod, 2007. 22(10): p. 2763-7.

956. Cai, L.Y., et al., *Abnormal placental cord insertion may induce intrauterine growth restriction in IVF-twin pregnancies.* Hum Reprod, 2006. 21(5): p. 1285-90.

957. Joo, J.G., et al., *Fetal pathology in second-trimester miscarriages.* Fetal Diagn Ther, 2009. 25(2): p. 186-91.

958. Cristina, M.P., et al., *Perinatal results following the prenatal ultrasound diagnosis of single umbilical artery.* Acta Obstet Gynecol Scand, 2005. 84(11): p. 1068-74.

959. Horton, A.L., L. Barroilhet, and H.M. Wolfe, *Perinatal Outcomes in Isolated Single Umbilical Artery.* Am J Perinatol, 2009.

960. Sikandar, R. and S. Munim, *Sirenomelia, the Mermaid syndrome: case report and a brief review of literature.* J Pak Med Assoc, 2009. 59(10): p. 721-3.

961. Jung, E., B.Y. Lee, and C.Y. Huh, *Prenatal diagnosis of fetal seizure: a case report.* J Korean Med Sci, 2008. 23(5): p. 906-8.

962. Bombrys, A.E., et al., *Pregnancy outcome in isolated single umbilical artery.* Am J Perinatol, 2008. 25(4): p. 239-42.

963. Gornall, A.S., J.J. Kurinczuk, and J.C. Konje, *Antenatal detection of a single umbilical artery: does it matter?* Prenat Diagn, 2003. 23(2): p. 117-23.

964. Dagklis, T., et al., *Isolated single umbilical artery and fetal karyotype.* Ultrasound Obstet Gynecol.

965. Rittler, M., et al., *SINGLE UMBILICAL ARTERY AND ASSOCIATED MALFORMATIONS IN OVER 5,500 AUTOPSIES. RELEVANCE FOR PERINATAL MANAGEMENT.* Pediatr Dev Pathol.

966. Burshtein, S., et al., *Is single umbilical artery an independent risk factor for perinatal mortality?* Arch Gynecol Obstet, 2009.

967. Hua, M., et al., *Single umbilical artery and its associated findings.* Obstet Gynecol. 115(5): p. 930-4.

968. Feinstein, S.J., et al., *Intrapartum ultrasound diagnosis of nuchal cord as a decisive factor in management.* Am J Obstet Gynecol, 1985. 153(3): p. 308-9.

969. Gracheva, T.I. and A.V. Mourachko, *Labour management in patients with pathology of the umbilical cord.* Frontiers in Fetal Health, 2001. 3: p. 129.

970. Zhang, H.X., X. Kong, and W.Y. Yang, *A case with a 137 cm long cord around the neck 6 times with bradycardia.* Chinese J Obstet Gynecol, 1990. 25: p. 161.

971. Gembruch, U. and A.A. Baschat, *True knot of the umbilical cord: transient constrictive effect to umbilical venous blood flow demonstrated by Doppler sonography.* Ultrasound Obstet Gynecol, 1996. 8(1): p. 53-6.

972. Vroonen, P. and J.P. Schaaps, *[Image of the month. Knotted umbilical cord]*. Rev Med Liege, 2000. 55(3): p. 154-5.

973. Gianopoulos, J., et al., *Diagnosis of vasa previa with ultrasonography.* Obstet Gynecol, 1987. 69(3 Pt 2): p. 488-91.

974. Hurley, V.A., *The antenatal diagnosis of vasa praevia: the role of ultrasound.* Aust N Z J Obstet Gynaecol, 1988. 28(3): p. 177-9.

975. Schellpfeffer, M.A., *Improved neonatal outcome of vasa previa with aggressive intrapartum management. A report of two cases.* J Reprod Med, 1995. 40(4): p. 327-32.

976. Catanzarite, V., et al., *Prenatal sonographic diagnosis of vasa previa: ultrasound findings and obstetric outcome in ten cases.* Ultrasound Obstet Gynecol, 2001. 18(2): p. 109-15.

977. Yampolsky, M., et al., *Centrality of the Umbilical Cord Insertion in a Human Placenta Influences the Placental Efficiency.* Placenta, 2009.

978. Eddleman, K.A., et al., *Clinical significance and sonographic diagnosis of velamentous umbilical cord insertion.* Am J Perinatol, 1992. 9(2): p. 123-6.

979. Sepulveda, W., et al., *True knot of the umbilical cord: a difficult prenatal ultrasonographic diagnosis.* Ultrasound Obstet Gynecol, 1995. 5(2): p. 106-8.

980. Challis, J.R. and S.K. Smith, *Fetal endocrine signals and preterm labor.* Biol Neonate, 2001. 79(3-4): p. 163-7.

981. Parry, A.J. and S. Westaby, *Cardiopulmonary bypass during pregnancy.* Ann Thorac Surg, 1996. 61(6): p. 1865-9.

982. Pirhonen, J.P. and R.U. Erkkola, *Uterine and umbilical flow velocity waveforms in the supine hypotensive syndrome.* Obstet Gynecol, 1990. 76(2): p. 176-9.

983. Dickey, R.P., *Doppler ultrasound investigation of uterine and ovarian blood flow in infertility and early pregnancy.* Hum Reprod Update, 1997. 3(5): p. 467-503.

984. Leible, S., et al., *Discordant uterine artery velocity waveforms as a predictor of subsequent miscarriage in early viable pregnancies.* Am J Obstet Gynecol, 1998. 179(6 Pt 1): p. 1587-93.

985. Hohmann, M., et al., *[Hypotonic symptoms and pregnancy].* Z Geburtshilfe Perinatol, 1992. 196(3): p. 118-22.

986. Mikheenko, G.A., *Myocardial contractility in pregnant women with arterial hypotension and its effect on the functional status of the fetus.* Akush Ginekol (Mosk), 1991. 1: p. 18-21.

987. Nakai, Y., et al., *Effects of maternal prone position on the umbilical arterial flow.* Acta Obstet Gynecol Scand, 1998. 77(10): p. 967-9.

988. Scheler, C. and F. Ropke, *[Blood flow in the umbilical artery in maternal hypotension and after therapy with Pholedrine longo--a Doppler ultrasound study].* Z Geburtshilfe Perinatol, 1993. 197(4): p. 191-4.

989. Brotanek, V., C.H. Hendricks, and T. Yoshida, *Changes in uterine blood flow during uterine contractions.* Am J Obstet Gynecol, 1969. 103(8): p. 1108-16.

990. Friedman, E.A. and R.K. Neff, *Hypertension-hypotension in pregnancy. Correlation with fetal outcome.* JAMA, 1978. 239(21): p. 2249-51.

991. Goeschen, K., *Bedeutung der orthostatischen Dysregulation in der Graviditat und unter der Gebut.* Hypotonie in der Schwangerschaft-Risiko oder Bagatelle, ed. K. Goeschen and J. Schneider. 1988, pp 18-23, Munchen: W. Zuckschwerdt Verlag.

992. Ng, P.H. and W.A. Walters, *The effects of chronic maternal hypotension during pregnancy.* Aust N Z J Obstet Gynaecol, 1992. 32(1): p. 14-6.

993. Christensen, E.C., K. Olsen, and W.F. Rayburn, *Increased patient acceptance and adherence using a new fetal movement chart.* Obstet Gynecol, 2001. 97: p. S38.

994. de Graaf, J.P., et al., *Increased adverse perinatal outcome of hospital delivery at night.* BJOG.

995. Gould, J.B., et al., *Neonatal mortality in weekend vs weekday births.* JAMA, 2003. 289(22): p. 2958-62.

996. Urato, A.C., et al., *The association between time of birth and fetal injury resulting in death.* Am J Obstet Gynecol, 2006. 195(6): p. 1521-6.

997. Caughey, A.B., et al., *Time of delivery and neonatal morbidity and mortality.* Am J Obstet Gynecol, 2008. 199(5): p. 496 e1-5.

998. Borruto, F., C. Comparetto, and A. Treisser, *Prevention of cerebral palsy during labour: role of foetal lactate.* Arch Gynecol Obstet, 2008. 278(1): p. 17-22.

999. Zhang, X., et al., *Prenatal and Perinatal Risk Factors for Autism in China.* J Autism Dev Disord.

1000. Gonzalez-Quintero, V.H., et al., *Outcomes of pregnancies with sonographically detected nuchal cords remote from delivery.* J Ultrasound Med, 2004. 23(1): p. 43-7.

1001. Sharkey, J.T., et al., *Melatonin synergizes with oxytocin to enhance contractility of human myometrial smooth muscle cells.* J Clin Endocrinol Metab, 2009. 94(2): p. 421-7.

1002. Hasegawa, J., *Studies for early identification of umbilical cord abnormalities and for management of high risk prengnancies with them.* ACta Obstet Gynaec Jpn, 2008. 60(9): p. 1723-1734.

1003. Saller, D.N., Jr., et al., *The clinical utility of the perinatal autopsy.* JAMA, 1995. 273(8): p. 663-5.

1004. Cunningham, F.G., et al., eds. *Williams Obstetrics (ed 21).* 2001. p 831-835, McGraw-Hill: N.Y., N.Y.

1005. Mvumbi, L., et al., *Decreased placental and umbilical cord glycogen levels associated with meconium-stained amniotic fluid.* Placenta, 1998. 16: p. 295-99.

1006. Mvumbi, L., et al., *Glycogen levels in human term placental disks, umbilical cords, and membranes.* Pediatr Pathol Lab Med, 1996. 16(4): p. 597-605.

1007. Collins, J.H., *Umbilical cord accidents: human studies.* Semin Perinatol, 2002. 26(1): p. 79-82.

1008. Meis, P.J., et al., *Variable decelerations during nonstress tests are not a sign of fetal compromise.* Am J Obstet Gynecol, 1986. 154(3): p. 586-90.

1009. Tita, A.T., et al., *Timing of elective repeat cesarean delivery at term and neonatal outcomes.* N Engl J Med, 2009. 360(2): p. 111-20.

1010. Bianchi, D.W., T.M. Crombleholme, and M.E. D'Alton, eds. *Fetology: Chapter 109 Umbilical-Cord Abnormalities.* 2000. p 822-825, McGraw-Hill: Philadelphia, PA.

1011. Deprest, J.A.M. and Y. Ville, *Obstetric Endoscopy*. The Unborn Patient, The Art and Science of Fetal Therapy, ed. M.R. Harrison, et al. 2001. p 213-31, Philadelphia, PA: W B Saunders.

1012. Caughey, A.B., et al., *Maternal and neonatal outcomes of elective induction of labor.* Evid Rep Technol Assess (Full Rep), 2009(176): p. 1-257.

1013. Darmstadt, G.L., et al., *Reducing stillbirths: interventions during labour.* BMC Pregnancy Childbirth, 2009. 9 Suppl 1: p. S6.

1014. Hodgson, E. and E. Norwitz, *Does low blood pressure increase the risk of stillbirth?*, in *Contemporary OB/GYN*. 2006, Contemporary OB/GYN.

1015. de Heus, R., et al., *The effects of the tocolytics atosiban and nifedipine on fetal movements, heart rate and blood flow.* J Matern Fetal Neonatal Med, 2009. 22(6): p. 485-90.

1016. de Heus, R., et al., *Adverse drug reactions to tocolytic treatment for preterm labour: prospective cohort study.* BMJ, 2009. 338: p. b744.

1017. Laohapojanart, N., et al., *Safety and efficacy of oral nifedipine versus terbutaline injection in preterm labor.* J Med Assoc Thai, 2007. 90(11): p. 2461-9.

1018. van Veen, A.J., et al., *Severe hypotension and fetal death due to tocolysis with nifedipine.* BJOG, 2005. 112(4): p. 509-10.

1019. Chan, L.W., et al., *Side-effect and vital sign profile of nifedipine as a tocolytic for preterm labour.* Hong Kong Med J, 2008. 14(4): p. 267-72.

1020. Johnson, K.A. and G.C. Mason, *Severe hypotension and fetal death due to tocolysis with nifedipine.* BJOG, 2005. 112(11): p. 1583.

1021. Kandysamy, V. and A.J. Thomson, *Severe hypotension and fetal death due to tocolysis with nifedipine.* BJOG, 2005. 112(11): p. 1583-4.

1022. Papatsonis, D.N., et al., *Severe hypotension and fetal death due to tocolysis with nifedipine.* BJOG, 2005. 112(11): p. 1582-3.

1023. van Geijn, H.P., J.E. Lenglet, and A.C. Bolte, *Nifedipine trials: effectiveness and safety aspects.* BJOG, 2005. 112 Suppl 1: p. 79-83.

1024. Erkinaro, T., et al., *Placental and fetal hemodynamics after labetalol or pindolol in a sheep model of increased placental vascular resistance and maternal hypertension.* Reprod Sci, 2009. 16(8): p. 749-57.

1025. Turton, P., et al., *Incidence, correlates and predictors of post-traumatic stress disorder in the pregnancy after stillbirth.* Br J Psychiatry, 2001. 178: p. 556-60.

1026. Samuelsson, M., I. Radestad, and K. Segesten, *A waste of life: fathers' experience of losing a child before birth.* Birth, 2001. 28(2): p. 124-30.

1027. Woods, J.R. and J.L. Woods, eds. *Loss During Pregnancy or in the Newborn Period.* 1997, Jannetti Publications: Pitman, NJ.

1028. Douglas, A., *Trying Again.* 2000, Dallas, TX: Taylor Publishing.

Ultrasound Review of the Umbilical Cord

Sonography of the umbilical cord..
Dudiak CM[1], Salomon CG, Posniak HV, Olson MC, Flisak ME
Radiographics. 1995 Sep;15(5):1035-50.

Sonographically detected abnormalities of the umbilical cord.
Shipp TD[1], Bromley B, Benacerraf BR.
Int J Gynaecol Obstet. 1995 Feb;48(2):179-85.

Prenatal ultrasonographic morphologic assessment of the umbilical cord: a review. Part I.
Sherer DM, Anyaegbunam A.
Obstet Gynecol Surv. 1997 Aug;52(8):506-14. Review.

Prenatal ultrasonographic morphologic assessment of the umbilical cord: a review. Part II.
Sherer DM, Anyaegbunam A.
Obstet Gynecol Surv. 1997 Aug;52(8):515-23. Review.

[The genetic sonogram].
Ben-Ami M, Jadaon JE.
Harefuah. 2009 Jul;148(7):455-9, 474. Review.

Comprehensive imaging review of abnormalities of the umbilical cord. Moshiri M1, Zaidi SF, Robinson TJ, Bhargava P, Siebert JR, Dubinsky TJ, Katz DS. Radiographics. 2014 Jan-Feb;34(1):179-96.

www.ingramcontent.com/pod-product-compliance
Lightning Source LLC
Chambersburg PA
CBHW030918180526
45163CB00002B/379